PLANT
SPIRIT
MEDICINE

PLANT SPIRIT MEDICINE

*A Journey into the
Healing Wisdom
of Plants*

ELIOT COWAN

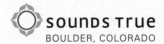
BOULDER, COLORADO

Sounds True, Inc.
Boulder, CO 80306

This work is solely for personal growth and education. It should not be treated as a substitute for psychotherapy or medical advice. In the event of physical or mental distress, please consult with appropriate health professionals.

Cover design by Rachael Murray
Book design by Beth Skelley

Printed in the United States of America

Library of Congress Cataloging-in-Publication Data

Cowan, Eliot, 1946–

Plant spirit medicine : a journey into the healing wisdom of plants / Eliot Cowan.

pages cm

ISBN 978-1-62203-095-8

1. Huichol Indians—Ethnobotany. 2. Huichol Indians—Medicine.
3. Huichol Indians—Religion. 4. Ethnobotany—Mexico.
5. Medicinal plants—Mexico. 6. Healing—Mexico.
7. Shamanism—Mexico. I. Title.

F1221.H9C69 2014

615.8'80972—dc23

2013037899

Ebook ISBN 978-1-62203-163-4

10 9 8 7 6

DEDICATED TO YOU.

MAY THE MEDICINE IN THESE PAGES
TOUCH YOUR HEART.

contents

acknowledgments

I spent a great many days gathering experience and putting words on these pages—days that might otherwise have been passed with my family. Victoria, Aura, Serena, Omar, and Vicky, I offer you love and thanks. May your patience and generosity be well rewarded.

Alison Gayek, you have worked tirelessly for many years as a magnificent teacher and champion of plant spirit medicine. Should the medicine continue to flourish, it will largely be thanks to you.

Ancestors and spirits of the Blue Deer Center, you favor this work in miraculous ways. You on the board and staff of the center have contributed more devotion, vision, skill, and hard work than anyone could expect. Thank you and thanks to all you generous friends of the center for giving the medicine and myself the perfect home.

Pam Meyer and Brian Crissey, you have my admiration and thanks for your loyalty to this book. You kept it in print for eighteen years and then gracefully sent it on to a new future.

Amy Rost and the other good people at Sounds True, you support *Plant Spirit Medicine* with taste, skill, and kindness.

Thank you, my brother Ish, for unfailing moral support.

I give astonished gratitude to you plant spirits for your generosity, wisdom, and healing.

To you plant spirit medicine students who give me hope
for the future,

To you healers who courageously offer this medicine
to a society that had forgotten it,

To you supporters of the Plant Spirit Medicine Association,

To the Temple of Sacred Fire Healing,

To you, Margaret Freier, pillar of the Temple,

May you be richly blessed by the divine natural world you serve so well.

You the God of Teachings and Lessons, God of Heart and Love, Knower of All Beings, Source and Keeper of Traditions, and true Author of this work, my stammering and insufficient thanks.

author's note

The stories of spiritual healing in this book are true, although names have been changed to respect the privacy of those who consulted me. For illustrative effect I have chosen unusually dramatic anecdotes; you should know that time, patience, and recurrence are needed to get the best that plant spirit medicine has to offer.

You should also know that plant spirit medicine does not diagnose, treat, or cure any physical, mental, or emotional symptom, condition, or illness. It provides purely spiritual intervention. No claims are made about changes in the health of those receiving treatment.

introduction

OUR WISEST ELDER

W hen I began writing this book in 1991, I had been practicing and teaching plant spirit medicine for a number
of years, and I had just begun an apprenticeship with a
Huichol Indian shaman in Mexico. I felt his medicine and mine were
both valuable because they promoted balance, even though most people I
knew didn't find balance very interesting at the time.

Back then it seemed the American way of life would go on forever.
There was some lip service being paid to sustainability, but few were *really*
concerned about it, and almost no one saw sustainability as having anything to do with spiritual healing. I was pretty much alone in my work,
stubbornly exploring new territory that turned out to be very old. Restor-
ing ancient ways of balance looked interesting to me in 1991. Today it
looks *necessary,* it looks urgent—and I no longer feel alone.

The loneliness is gone largely because this small book brought many
extraordinary people to be my students. Some of them became plant spirit
medicine healers, some engaged with Huichol shamanism, and some
explored and discovered other paths. Many are working today to make
life satisfying and sustainable once again. Their good-hearted work is producing important changes. When I wrote the first edition of this book,

for example, I pointed out that our young people did not have effective rituals of initiation into adulthood. I mentioned some of the resulting illnesses and sufferings, but I could offer no remedy. Today, thanks to the Sacred Fire Community, authentic initiation is once more available.

At the same time, much has been lost. Violence upon human beings and the natural world has escalated, while the keepers of wisdom have become an endangered species. Only a few years ago indigenous leaders and medicine people in the Peruvian Amazon were slaughtered by heavily armed police while attempting to save their forest homeland from corporate development. Sadly, this is far from an isolated case; the genocide of heart-centered people goes on throughout the "undeveloped" world, while the "developed" world becomes more aggressive as it falters and fails.

Where loss of habitat and outright murder are less intense, age and illness are claiming the wise elders. Most of the teachers I write about in this book are now gone. The great Huichol shaman don José Ríos (Matsuwa) died in 1990 at 110 years of age. Don Guadalupe González Ríos, with whom I apprenticed, died in 2003. The preeminent English acupuncturist, Professor J. R. Worsley—my guide to the Five Elements—died the same year. Don José Benítez Sánchez, the Huichol artist and shaman who introduced me to don Guadalupe, passed away in 2008. The warm and funny Ute medicine woman Grandma Bertha Grove left this world in 2009.

Don Lucio Campos Elizalde, the weather shaman and healer, passed away in 2005 at ninety-three years of age. An outline of his life might give some feeling for what the world loses with the death of such an elder and what hope and guidance he leaves behind.

Don Lucio was born, lived, and died in the tiny village of Nepopualco, Morelos, in the central highlands of Mexico. He was a Nahua Indian. As a young man, he used to make long journeys on foot to the city in order to hear Spanish spoken. In this way he taught himself to be fluent in that language. His people were campesinos, or peasants, and don Lucio continued to raise crops and livestock throughout his life. In his early twenties he was struck by lightning. He fell into a coma and was in and out of that state for three years. The first year he spent traveling and learning in the realm of the weather beings: rain, wind, cloud, sun, ocean, and certain mountain beings, as well as their commanding Great Goddess, whom he called Santa Barbarita. The second year he dwelled with the plant spirits, and the third year he spent with the animal spirits. He emerged from those years as a man of knowledge and wisdom, which he shared generously with his people for the rest of his life. He had become an extraordinary healer, and his gifts benefited many people.

Don Lucio was especially devoted to Santa Barbarita, who gave him the task of helping people maintain a good relationship with the sacred weather beings in order to ensure beneficial weather for crops, animals, and humans. He applied himself to the instructions of the Goddess and became an important leader of traditional rituals related to weather. He identified and initiated many people who were themselves called to become "weather workers," and he guided and supported them in their work. One result of their efforts was the unusually stable and beneficial weather patterns in that part of Mexico.

Toward the end of his life, don Lucio initiated David Wiley, an American living nearby in Mexico, into weather work. David showed exceptional promise; the older man made him the organizational leader for the group of non-Mexican weather workers who had gathered around don Lucio. This group was well loved by don Lucio, for they were the hardest working and most devoted to their path. In time, there were more foreigners than Mexicans under Lucio's guidance. After ceremonies in Nepopualco, they would return to their homes and work to restore balance between their communities and the weather beings. In this way, important but long-neglected relationships began to be revived and restored.

Just before his death, don Lucio imparted to David Wiley special knowledge and blessings and made him his successor. Under don David's care, the weather-work fraternity continues to grow and benefit many communities.

As wisdom keepers like don Lucio die, the cloak of elderhood is passed on to people of my generation—a generation born and raised in a society entranced by youth and uninterested in wisdom. Today our way of life is collapsing under the weight of its own greed; the need for wise elders has never been greater, yet there has perhaps never been a generation less prepared to provide wisdom.

Somehow, miraculously, the cloak is put on and wisdom reappears: A don Lucio sees fertile ground in the soul of a David Wiley. The soil is cultivated, and since the old man's death, a conventional American business consultant grows into a wise elder himself. In a few years, the younger man tends a flourishing of the tradition such as the older man had not seen in his long lifetime.

One function of an elder is to demonstrate the wisdom of our wisest elder: the natural world itself. I say "demonstrate" because talk is not enough. I can say, "The natural world sustains itself with balanced relationships, and it can also restore balance, healing, and sustainability in human life." This may sound appealing, but as an idea it is soon drowned out in the din of other ideas clamoring for attention. Even if you agree with it, nothing will have changed from thinking about it. An experience, on the other hand, can be denied and even forgotten, but it cannot be unexperienced. Experience changes you forever.

When your heart is touched by the medicine of a plant spirit, you *feel* the love and wisdom of the natural world. Ideas do not deliver the same touch; therefore, this book is not a theoretical treatise or a how-to manual. Mostly this is a book of stories, because stories aim for the heart, where experience lives.

Plant spirit medicine works partially because it has broad perspective. It does not look only through the eyes of physics and chemistry; it sees human beings as expressions of divine natural forces. It plumbs the human mind and emotions. It gives paramount importance to spirit, the mysterious core of our lives.

My apprenticeship, initiation, and work as a *marakame,* or shaman in the Huichol tradition, steeped me in a perspective larger than the one I had in 1991. I find myself now with even deeper appreciation for the medicine of the plant spirits, and I've tried to share that appreciation with you. While Huichol shamanism is not the subject of this new edition of *Plant Spirit Medicine,* the shamanic perspective brought forth new chapters and improved the older ones. I trust you will feel enriched by it as I have, seeing how this mysterious healing weaves into our relationships with ourselves, our loved ones, community, ancestors, worldview, and the forces of the divine natural world.

By way of tipping my hat in respect, I will mention that the Huichols are an indigenous people whose once-extensive homelands have been reduced to some rugged areas in the western Sierra Madre in the states of Jalisco, Nayarit, and Durango, Mexico. Like all indigenous peoples in the Western Hemisphere, the Huichols have been and are being hard pressed by the dominant culture. Unlike most indigenous groups, though, they have never been conquered, they have not converted to foreign religions, they have not lost their language, their communities are functional, and their ancestral spiritual traditions are still robust. This is not to say that life in a Huichol village is idyllic. The people face many problems: they have few possessions, scanty modern education, little money, and no reliable friends in high places to protect them from the predators who circle around their natural resources. Even though their lives are hard, the Huichol know who they are, where they are, and what is important. Their world is not a world of inert "things"; it is a living world of divine feeling and expression. They live in a mood of restrained joy mostly unknown to Western people.

Like Huichol medicine, plant spirit medicine is low tech; it produces healing purely through good relationship with the natural world. In this way it is not simply a relic of the past; it is also a medicine for the present and the future. Whether you consider high technology a blessing or a curse, we are now confronting this reality: the world cannot support the extraction of resources; production of heat; and contamination of air, water, and soil necessary to build machines and keep them running. High-tech medicine is already too expensive for most of humanity. Like everything unsustainable, it is destined to become more extravagant and rare until there is a collapse of the unbalanced system that props it up.

No doubt collapse will produce hardship and even tragedy, but it will also bring us back to what traditional healers and indigenous elders have always demonstrated: plants, animals, rocks, water, fire, wind, and the entire natural world know us and love us as grandchildren. We don't have to steal from them because they have what we require, and they are glad to give it to us. We are just asked to follow a simple rule: take only what you need and give back something that satisfies the one you've taken from.

These pages open to the medicine dream of the natural world. It is a big dream; all plants live there. You and I live there too.

How do we get to the medicine of the dream? How does it work? What exactly is it anyway? You will find some information here, but explanation is not my task. My hope is that this book may be the medicine. And my prayer is that it may touch you as you read.

part one

PLANTS, SPIRITS, AND THEIR MEDICINE

chapter 1

Plant Spirit Medicine Dreams

The American adventurer Peter Gorman is walking down a trail in the Amazon jungle. He is on his way back to the village after watching his Matsés Indian friend set a trap for wild boar. The Indian takes advantage of the walk to show Peter some medicinal plants growing along the trail. Within a few minutes, he has pointed out several dozen species and pantomimed their healing virtues.

Arriving at the village, Peter summons his interpreter and returns to the hunter's hut. He didn't have his notebook with him on the walk, he explains, and he couldn't possibly remember all he had been shown. Would the hunter be kind enough to say once again how the herbs were prepared and used?

The hunter-shaman smiles at Peter and then begins to laugh. He invites all his wives and children over to have a good laugh, too. When they have all laughed themselves out, he explains, "That was just to introduce you to some of the plants. If you want to actually use a plant yourself, the spirit of the plant must come to you in your dreams. If the spirit of the plant tells you how to prepare it and what it will cure, you can use it. Otherwise, it won't work for you. That was a good one! I've got to remember what you just said!" He laughs again.

Meanwhile, in Connecticut, a major pharmaceutical firm approaches a shamanic studies institute. The firm wants to contact shamans of the Amazon in order to get information on medicinal plants. The company plans to take samples of the herbs, isolate active molecules, and manufacture them in the laboratory.

I can imagine the scene when the pharmaceutical firm makes it to the Amazon: The shamans laughing uproariously as they collect their meager fees. The field workers rushing specimens back to the laboratory. Skilled technicians spending millions of company dollars researching new compounds, only to come up with one disappointment after another. The shamans will be discredited, but they won't care. They will still be in the jungle, working cures with the plants they have used for centuries.

The American firm, infatuated with its "superior" technology, will go to the jungle dreaming of profits from a patentable new drug. No one will think of asking the shamans what the active ingredients are. If they do ask, they won't like the answer. There is only one active ingredient in plant medicines: friendship. A plant spirit heals a patient as a favor to its friend-in-dreaming, the doctor.

To the people of the Amazon this truth is basic. Any four-year-old understands it. That is why the Matsés hunter-shaman called his children over to have a good laugh at Peter. They couldn't believe a grown man could be so silly!

The Matsés and many other non-European peoples understand that both nature and humankind are endowed with awareness and spirit. Therefore, humans and nature are of the same family. In all cultures there exist individuals who have especially vivid experiences with the spirits of nature. When properly trained and initiated, these people become shamans. Shamans make friends of the spirits of nature and call upon them for help with everyday affairs.

Plant spirit medicine is the shaman's way with plants. It recognizes that plants have spirit and that spirit is the strongest medicine. Spirit can heal the deepest reaches of the heart and soul.

There is nothing exotic about all this. Don't be misled by talk about the Amazon. If you want to meet the most powerful healing plants in the world, just open your door and step outside. They are growing all around you. If you don't believe me, or if you have a taste for romantic locations, you can try going elsewhere. But if you stay there long enough, it comes down to the same thing: dealing with the local weeds.

In keeping with this homegrown quality, I want to tell you what was happening around my home as I wrote this chapter. At first this may seem to have nothing to do with our subject, but bear with me; in time it will make sense.

I went to visit a Huichol Indian named José Benítez Sánchez. In certain circles, José was famous as a visionary artist. Among his own people he was known as a shaman. José lived part time in a village near Tepic, Mexico. The rest of the time he lived in the resort city of Puerto Vallarta. It was there I went to find him.

As I approached his home in one of the humblest districts in town, I recalled the first time I'd met José, the year before. This was a man who earned a huge income by Indian standards. Yet as he welcomed me into his house, it was apparent that he had but one material possession of any consequence—an electric fan. Our visit was brief, for he was due to leave in a few hours to meet with the president of Mexico.

José cheerfully admitted that he did not have money for bus fare. Looking down at his ragged cutoffs, he allowed that he also did not own a pair of pants to wear to greet the president. Evidently he sensed I was confused about why a successful man should be so destitute, for he told me the following story:

> When I was a boy, I admired my grandfather. He was a powerful
> shaman. One day when he felt I was old enough to understand,
> he told me, "José, there are two types of power that one can
> acquire. One type is used for your own personal reasons. The
> other is used for the benefit of your people. You can walk the road
> to the first type of power or to the second. But let me tell you this:
> the second road is the road to happiness." Because my grandfather
> was a very wise man, I took his advice, and I have stayed on the
> second road. Whenever the gods give me something, I immedi-
> ately pass it on for the use of my people.

José's presence radiated contentment. Obviously his grandfather had known what he was talking about. I dug into my suitcase and came up with a pair of pants, which I presented to him, together with his bus fare. He accepted my gifts with sincere thanks and not a trace of surprise. Then he took off on his voyage to see the president, leaving me one small step farther down the road to happiness.

As I was reminiscing about that first meeting, I looked up to see José walking toward me. José was a good-looking, compact man of middle years. That day he was wearing long pants, a short-sleeved shirt, and a cowboy hat. The only sign of his background was his intensely colorful Huichol shoulder bag. He invited me into his house, and we sat down at a table with two of his paintings-in-progress. We chatted about the pilgrimage he would be leading in a few days. Children toddled in and out. A teenage girl stood outside, her chin propped on the windowsill, listening carefully. Eventually I got around to the purpose of my visit.

"I want to ask your advice about something, don José."

"Of course. Go ahead."

"Did you know an old man, a great shaman named don José Ríos? They called him Matsuwa."

"Matsuwa, yes. He was a relative of mine."

"Well, I met him years ago, and he helped me. Then, about three years ago, my father was dying of cancer. He said he wanted a shaman to help him, so I went to see Matsuwa. He was living in Las Blancas at that time."

José nodded.

"When I arrived, I found that Matsuwa was as bad off as my father was. He was very weak and couldn't get out of bed. He was moaning with pain; he said that his legs were killing him. He was lying in the hot sun, but he was shivering with cold. I had to put a blanket over him."

José made a face to let me know he understood the anguish of the moment.

"It occurred to me to see if I could help Matsuwa. I gave him a treatment. Right away he stopped shivering and asked to have the blanket taken off. His legs stopped hurting too, although he was still too weak to sit up. When the people saw this, they asked me if I could help them too. One of Matsuwa's nephews took me to see his father, who had been hit by a train and couldn't walk. On the way to see his father, the boy asked me if I believed in the Huichol way of healing, using feathers. I said, yes, of course I believed in it. 'In fact,' I told him, 'your uncle helped me a lot with his feathers. I would like to learn about Huichol healing myself.'

"The boy told me that there was someone in the village who was very good at healing with feathers. This man had learned his skill by making a pilgrimage every year for five years to a nearby peak."

"That peak is called 'El Picacho,'" said José.

"You know it, then," I said.

"Of course."

"Well, after that I returned to the United States, and I began to visit El Picacho in my dreams. I want to tell you what I saw in my dreams, so that you can advise me, don José."

"What did you see?" José asked me.

"At the very top of the mountain there is a flat area where two trees grow. There is a person there, a Huichol man. He is short. His face is round; he has plump cheeks. He smiles all the time. The little man is accompanied by a small deer. The deer dances and does all sorts of antics. The deer and the man let me know that they can help me to heal people.

"I have dreamed of this place many times now. There have been occasions when people who live far away have asked me to heal them. Because I didn't know what else to do, I asked the man and the deer to do the work. There have been some very good results."

"It is exactly as you say," said José.

"What do you mean?" I asked.

"The tree you saw is the Wind Tree that grows on that peak. The short man lives there too. He is the magic of the Wind Tree. If you go there he will talk to you, just as we are talking. But you should tell him to talk with you in Spanish, because you don't understand Huichol.

"I have seen this little Huichol man. He crosses my path when I am on pilgrimage to visit the gods. I ask his permission to pass. I explain that I am on my way to someplace else, and he lets me go. Just as you say, he is very short and has fat cheeks and thick lips. Actually, he is very, very old, although often he appears to be young. The deer lives there at El Picacho as well. Sometimes the antlers of the deer appear on the head of the little man. This is all the magic of the Wind Tree, which you also saw in your dream. The Wind Tree teaches people how to heal. It also teaches music. There is a world-famous musician in our tribe. It was the Wind Tree that taught him."

I said, "You tell me that a Wind Tree grows on the peak, but there were two trees in my vision."

"They are both the Wind Tree," José replied. "One represents the left antlers of the deer and the other represents the right antlers. Many people go and make the sacrifice to the Wind Tree there at El Picacho. This is a very good thing. Because you have dreamed this, it would be very good for you to go. The little man you saw does live there. If you go with faith and ask that he appear to you so that you can learn from him, he will appear in person.

"However, it would be necessary to consult first with someone who is familiar with the magic of El Picacho, someone who has made the sacrifice. I myself rarely go to that region. I keep busy with other sacrifices, other pilgrimages. There is someone in my village, though, who knows the mountain very well. His name is Guadalupe González Ríos, and he is also related to José Ríos. He is a very good man, not at all stingy with information. I am going to our village tomorrow. When I see him, immediately I will remember this conversation, and I will tell him about you. Perhaps you can come to the *fiesta* when we return from our pilgrimage. The three of us can talk together then. We should be back by the twenty-fourth."

"What day of the week is that?"

"Thursday, I believe."

"Friday!" said the girl in the window. This was her first contribution to the conversation.

"Too bad!" I said. "I will be in the United States at that time."

"Never mind. Come by my house when you return, and we will go to my village together. Perhaps I will bring along another man who has also dreamed of the Wind Tree. He is a German."

"Frenchman," chimed the girl.

More than once during my school years, I awoke in the middle of the night with the solution to a mathematical equation that had completely stumped me during the day. I never told anyone that I had done my algebra homework in my sleep. I was afraid that people would think I was weird. Eventually I stopped having these dreams.

Much later in life I discovered that it is not at all unusual for people to learn from dreams. Nowadays I enjoy asking people if they have ever dreamed something that later came to pass. About 75 percent say they have indeed had a dream of this type. And everyone has dreams that take place somewhere other than the bedroom where their sleeping body lies. When we dream, we can easily travel to distant places. We can know the future. We are given special understanding that enables us to solve life's problems.

For the most part, these wonderful dream powers lie dormant in our society, but the Huichols and the Matsés of the Amazon consider dream learning to be true learning. Indeed, nearly every culture on earth, except our own, respects dream learning as true learning. We revere the rational, analytical method of learning that has been honed and polished since the days of the ancient Greeks. We do not realize that the shamans of our species have honed and polished another method. This dreaming method is neither rational nor analytical, but it works extremely well.

The key to this method is to get into the dream state of consciousness, keeping in mind what it is that you wish to learn or accomplish. The way you get into the dream state is incidental. Some shamans learn to go to sleep and dream about what they wish to dream about. Others use psychotropic plants. Many simply listen to monotonous drumming to induce the dream state.

When I first heard about El Picacho several years ago, I was eager to learn from the spirits said to dwell there. With the demands of conducting a busy acupuncture practice, raising young children, and attending my dying father, it was impossible for me to visit the peak in person, so I decided to visit in dreams. (At that time I was not aware that it could be dangerous to engage a sacred site this way.) I lit a candle and some incense to help set the mood, then I lay down on my back and relaxed. I affirmed my intention to visit the sacred site and meet any helpful spirits that might live there. As I listened to loud, repetitive drumbeats, my state of consciousness shifted. My dream helpers appeared to me and flew me to the peak, where I had the experiences I recounted to José Benítez Sánchez during my current visit, several years after the original dream.

My conversation with José confirmed that my dream corresponded with an ancient tradition. As a Huichol and a shaman, he had no trouble accepting that I had met a tree spirit who could help me heal people. Being a middle-class white American, on the other hand, I have been plagued for years with the question, "Am I making this up?"

This is the question—the monster—faced by every Westerner who ventures into the world of dreams. There is only one way to subdue this monster: put the dream to the test and see if it works. If the magic of the Wind Tree can heal people, does it really matter whether I am making it up?

Several years ago, I guided a group of my students to dream the medicine of the willow. We were sitting in a circle, sharing our dreams. One man, a physician, said that there was an aspect of his dream he did not know how to interpret. "Over and over again," he said, "the willow spirit kept repeating to me, 'Look up! Look up! Always look up!'"

A month later I again met with the physician, who told the following story:

I have a patient who seemed perfect for willow medicine, so I've given it to her three times now. When she came back after the first treatment, she insisted I tell her what that "wonderful medicine" was. At the same time, she kept turning to a potted willow on my windowsill. She said something strange and wonderful: "That plant is so lovely. I would like to be that plant!"

I asked the woman to tell me what the treatment had done for her, and she mentioned improvements in a long list of physical complaints. "But," she said, "this is the best thing of all. I didn't realize it before, but I have been depressed all my life. I was so negative! It was as if my mind's eye was always looking down at the ground, and all I could see was the dirt. But you know, from the moment I left here last time, I heard a voice inside that said, 'Look up! Look up! Always look up!' and now it's as if I am seeing the beauty around me for the first time!"

At that moment I told her that the plant on the windowsill and the medicine she had taken were both willow. I also shared with her my willow dream and said I had heard the same voice saying, "Look up!" She was so moved she began to cry. At the next treatment she brought in a poem she had written to thank the willow spirit.

The experiences of the class, the physician, the patient—where did they come from? Is there such a thing as a willow spirit? If so, what is it really? Does it matter? Evidently it *did* matter to the young physician. Despite his experience with the willow spirit and his depressed patient, he decided that we were all just making it up, and he stopped practicing plant spirit medicine.

As for me, it seems that plant spirit medicine keeps practicing me. I thought I would go to José Benítez Sánchez and find out about an entirely different kind of healing having to do with sacred mountains, dancing deer, and such. I instead found out it is all about the magic of the Wind Tree. So I'm still learning medicine from plants.

chapter 2

PLANTS

The year is 1970. I am an urban expatriate trying to live on the land in northern Vermont. It is early spring; there is still snow on the ground. Soon it will be time to fix the fence, and I need posts. I shoulder a bow saw and a machete and set off to my favorite part of the farm—the cedar bog that surrounds the waterfall.

The sun is shining brightly today, although the air is still cool. As I enter the woods, I listen to the wind sifting through the cedar boughs. I take a pinch of leaves, crush them under my nose, and nod a greeting to the trees. The cedars here grow in little families, with several trunks sharing their roots. Among these families are miniature meadows, soon to be filled with grasses and wildflowers. I will spend the next two or three days working in this place. Had I brought the chainsaw, I could have been finished by lunchtime today—dinner at the latest. I make a mental note never to bring the chainsaw.

I have never cut fence posts by myself before. This time I can do it any way I want. How do I want to do it? If I were a tree growing here in this bog, how would I want it done?

I turn to the nearest cedar and ask it how I should cut the fence posts. I don't expect an answer, of course, and I don't get one.

Or do I?

Somehow it is now perfectly obvious how I will cut my posts. From each clump I will select a trunk that is crowding the others. I will carefully cut that trunk, limb it, and pile the brush on top of the stump. This way, I won't kill a single tree, I won't choke the meadows with brush piles, and I will leave the grove healthier and more beautiful than I found it. This will probably take me an extra day or so, but who cares?

Poet Gary Snyder said the way we kill our farm animals is a source of endless bad luck for our society. This is an interesting statement and, I think, a true one. It is based on an understanding of what in the East is called the law of karma. Here in the West, we express the same understanding through homilies: "What goes around, comes around." "He who lives by the sword shall die by the sword." Many people have expressed concern and even outrage at the unnatural and cruel lives and deaths inflicted upon our livestock. It took Snyder, who is no vegetarian, to point out that our behavior toward animals rebounds on us just like all the rest of our behavior. If we take lives without respect and gratitude for the sacrificed animals, then we too will be subject to humiliation and alienation. This is not cruel fate or harsh nature, but just us creating our own bad luck.

Might it not be also worthwhile to consider our relationship to plants? The most striking thing about this relationship is that we need them, but they don't need us. We humans are utterly dependent on plants to cover all our needs: fuel, shelter, clothing, medicine, the petrochemical cornucopia, and, of course, food. (Even meat is made of plants.) In contrast, plant communities do just fine without people. We seem to offer plants nothing but suffering, destruction, and the threat of extinction.

There is some karmic rebound here. We are devastating forests and the foundations of vegetable life: soil, air, water, and solar radiation. This is not only murderous, but also suicidal. Under the circumstances, the continued generosity of plants toward our species is absolutely remarkable. What makes plants so generous? What makes us so brutal?

Somewhere along the way, we lost the experience of unity. We live our lives propping up the pathetic lie that we are different from everything else. This is a lie because the same awareness shines in the heart of all things. The lie is pathetic because it dooms us to a dry life of alienation.

Difference breeds indifference. If you think the forest is not you, you are more willing to exploit it or let others exploit it for you.

Plants, on the other hand, are not under the illusion that they are separate from the rest of creation. Observe how any plant interacts with soil, air, minerals, animals, and insects. Everything around it is enriched and benefited by its presence. Plants live in harmony with nature. One might even say that plants *are* nature. Out of this union comes their incredible generosity to us and to all their other fellow creatures.

For the first time, I am dreaming with a plant. English plantain is growing here, and I see a young woman with enormous wings sprouting from her shoulders. Somehow I know she is the plantain spirit. I approach her and introduce myself. She asks why I have come.

"First of all," I reply, "I want to thank you for the help you have given my friends and me over the years. Your leaves have healed many wounds. I come to you to ask for another kind of help, a deeper kind. The cuts and scrapes of my people are nothing compared to the pain in our hearts and the pollution in our minds. Can you help relieve this kind of suffering too?"

The plantain woman hops off her leaf and flies close to me. For a moment she hovers in front of my face and looks intently into my eyes. Then she smiles and says, "Of course, I will help you. My brothers and sisters will help you also. We are very happy to do this. In fact, we have been waiting for two hundred years for someone to ask us for this kind of help. We can do nothing unless we are asked."

"We can do nothing unless we are asked." Leave it to a plant to come up with the understatement of the millennium!

Look at what plants do when they are asked: all human civilization is a form of excess grain—the generosity of plants. The history of our species shows us that plants furnish us with whatever we ask for. Our society values comfort, so that is what we have gone to the plant world to get.

Comfort is wonderful, as far as it goes—which is not very far in the direction of satisfaction. If for a moment we could forget the quest for comfort and ask plants to help us find joy, richness, and significance in life, is there any reason to suppose they would not share those qualities with us just as they have shared everything else?

All things enjoy ecstatic union with nature. Life without ecstasy is not true life and not worth living. Without ecstasy, the soul becomes shriveled and perverted, the mind becomes corrupt, and the body suffers pain. Ecstatic union with nature is necessary for normal health; it is necessary for survival. And to think that plants are mere dumb creatures that do not know ecstasy is ignorance or tragic, arrogant folly.

I once gave a class in which the students brought patients for me to treat. One of the patients was a middle-aged man just out of the hospital. He suffered from leukemia and had had a close brush with death. He had abandoned his artistic career and was wandering about looking for a treatment that could spare him pain in his last days. A dream journey to his soul revealed an inner landscape barren and forlorn as the most forbidding desert. I treated this man with the spirits of two plants. A few days later, I returned home. Before long, I got this letter from the student who followed up on this man's treatment:

> The man we saw earlier this month who had leukemia called me this week saying he had felt good results from the treatment and wanted to come see me for another treatment. When he came, he began to tell me what had happened to him. The day following your treatment with him, he awoke in what he called "a different state of consciousness," which has been constantly with him ever since. He spoke of "recollecting himself" by going to an island where his family had spent a lot of time, and also to a petroglyph that was an important rock to him and [that] had at one time spoken to him.
>
> Last week, [the man's] doctor reduced his white-cell-killing drug by half because his white cell count had dropped by half. The man cleaned up his studio and has begun painting again. He has been having what he calls "lucid dreams," and he speaks of the healing quality of these dreams.

Anticipating his treatment, I had decided to use the mullein spirit with him. The day before he arrived, I found mullein growing in a ravine. The following morning before he got to my house, I made another dream journey to the mullein. I was transported to a place where a crow waited for me alongside a colony of mullein plants. Nearby, a tree was standing. Among its limbs, crow feathers and mullein leaves formed a nest. Here someone [who] need[ed] nurturing would be fulfilled with waves of blessings. When [that person] was ready, [the crow] would then fly away.

When our patient arrived, I treated him with the mullein spirit. As he was lying on the table, he heard a crow outside my window. He began telling a story of having taken a baby crow that was once given to a girlfriend of his . . . [O]ur patient made a nest for it and cared for it for months. He spoke of how deeply he became involved, learning the ways of crows. When the time came, the crow he had cared for flew away.

The most remarkable thing in this story is that the patient entered a "different state of consciousness." This new consciousness enabled him to find healing in his dreams and allowed him to re-enter the magical connection with nature he'd had in his youth. Inside that magic, life was once again worth living, and the man's body responded by rallying to fight his disease. The proof that he was healed was that he cleaned up his studio and began to paint once again. In other words, he was resurrected. He came back to life.

Thanks to ecstatic union with nature, this man gained some chance of survival, whereas before he had none. Ultimately, though, healing is not about whether you die. Healing is about how fully you live. I hope this artist went on to live a long and fruitful life, but regardless of when he died, he would still be a great success, because he really lived.

For my protection and your enlightenment, it is worth making sure this is clear: I did *not* diagnose or treat this man for leukemia. Plant spirit medicine does not diagnose or treat any illness. I do not offer any herbal treatment as a cure for any disease. In a later chapter I will explain how the practitioner of plant spirit medicine, in assessing which plants to use with a given person, pays no attention whatsoever to any symptoms that person may have.

There are many examples of plants' willingness to reintroduce us to the joy of a close relationship with nature. A sixteen-year-old boy, for example, came to see me complaining of severe hay fever. Because he worked part time as a gardener, this was a serious handicap. After his first treatment, he returned and asked me what was that "weird stuff" I had given him. I asked him why he thought it was weird, and he replied, "On my way home from your office, all the trees and shrubs were, like, waving at me and stuff!" I knew immediately that the plants were signaling their friendliness to him and that their pollen would no longer cause him any trouble. This turned out to be true.

Other people have returned after treatment to tell me stories of "falling in love with the earth," or "feeling like I'm not alone," or "seeing fairies in my back yard." One of my favorite stories involves Karen, a woman in her twenties who was suffering from depression and a number of physical complaints. I chose to treat her with the spirit of hummingbird sage, a beautiful shrub that grows in the coastal ranges of Southern California, where I was living at the time. In my dream work with the hummingbird sage, the spirit appeared to me as a jolly, muscular little man full of fun and kindness. He was dressed in a pointed cap, a medieval tunic, leggings, and shoes with pointy, turned-up toes.

This was Karen's report after her treatment:

After I left here, I felt so tired that I went home and lay down. I was half asleep and had a dream or a daydream. It was totally vivid and lifelike. In this dream, I felt that someone else was entering my body. I wasn't frightened because I felt he was a very good person: kind and fun loving. I could see him very clearly. He was short and strong, and he wore funny old-fashioned clothing and shoes with pointy, turned-up toes. I felt he was there to give me something I needed.

That afternoon I felt a strong urge to go to my special spot in the mountains. There is a certain place I go: the smell there reminds me of the smell of the sage that grows in Colorado, in the Rockies. I lived in Colorado until my mother died. I guess I'm trying to recapture the feeling about life that I used to have when my mother was alive, so I go to this place. The problem is, I never

quite manage to get the feeling back. I get a little glimpse of it,
but it fades away. But this time, after the treatment, I went to my
spot, and it worked! I got that wonderful feeling back! In fact, it
still hasn't left me!

I asked Karen to draw me a detailed map of her special spot in the mountains. After work, I drove up and hiked to the exact location. There I found
one of the largest stands of the fragrant hummingbird sage I'd ever seen.

Some people, like Karen, are sensitive to these experiences and communicate them well. Others are less sensitive, less articulate. Many people
probably never tell me about them because they don't want me to think
they are crazy. I now believe that everyone who is touched by the plant
spirits gets some taste of magic and union with nature. The following is
an excerpt from a letter written by another observant, expressive woman
about the effects of her first treatment:

It was wonderful. No, better than that—it was fantastic, magical,
incredible, and, to top it all, you (or rather the spirits) cured me
of a deep and dark longing that I have carried with me like a pain
all my life. I feel that something has become clearer, has settled,
is no longer a question or a separation. Since I last saw you,
many strange and magical things have happened to me: dreams
and unusual coincidences. All of it confirms what I have always
believed—that everything is connected; all are part of the whole.
I have always known this but did not directly experience it. Since
your treatment, it's as if many doors have been pulled open and
the spirit allowed to rush in. I feel "touched," connected, whole,
and a little mad—intoxicated, full of joy!

Plants wish us well in every way. They are perfectly willing to bring us into
the blessings of their union with nature. But, as the plantain spirit told
me, they can do nothing unless they are asked. I would add that we have
to know the right questions and the right way to ask them.

What is the right way to ask a plant? Part of it has to do with appre-
ciating that a plant has roots. A plant lives in a particular location, with
its dirt, rain, sunshine, and air. With these particular elements it does its
growth magic. From plants we learn that if you want to enter nature, you

have to do it where you are, because that is the only place nature can be found. It follows that if you are going to ask a plant to bring you into the blessing of nature, it is best to ask a plant that lives where you live. The great English acupuncturist J. R. Worsley said, "Local herbs are not ten times stronger, not a hundred times stronger. Local herbs are *one thousand times* stronger than exotic ones!" Professor Worsley was not exaggerating.

One woman described her first treatment with (local) plant spirit medicine as "bringing me back to a place I've never been before." I puzzled over her words. How could she return to a place she had never been? Finally I got the sense of it. We are part of nature, but how many of us really *live* in nature? Whether we reside in mud huts or skyscrapers is not the point. The point is the joy of being in the dance of creation as an equal partner with everything. This means bringing us back to where we already live: on the earth, with the dirt, the rain, the sunshine, and the air—just like our brothers and sisters, the plants.

After her first plant spirit medicine treatment, Glenda, one of my patients, said that for two weeks she felt she was on the verge of receiving some sort of "spiritual message." At the second session I gave her mountain mahogany. The spirit of this plant appears to me as a wise old Native American Grandmother who comes from a tribe that performs ceremonies in underground chambers. I was hoping this Grandmother would be able to give Glenda the instruction she needed, for Grandmothers are guardians and teachers of traditional spiritual lore.

After the mountain mahogany treatment, Glenda started to hear two words, "Second Mesa," repeating in her head. She had never heard them together and had no idea what they meant. The following day, she and her husband were watching a television documentary on the Hopi Indians, and they both found it very interesting. After it was over, Glenda turned to her husband and said, "That's it—the Hopis! Someone there has the message for me. Darling, we've got to visit the Hopis!"

"Fine, dear, but where will we go? I don't know where the Hopis live, do you?"

"How am I supposed to know? I've never been out of California in my life!"

"Well, I'll get the road atlas. I think I heard that they live somewhere in Arizona."

The two of them pored over the map of Arizona and sure enough, there was the Hopi reservation. They looked closer.

"There it is: Second Mesa! Look, it's a village on the Hopi reservation! Next weekend we're gonna go to Second Mesa!"

When Friday came around, the other secretaries at Glenda's office were out sick, and she felt she couldn't take off time to go to Second Mesa. She was crushed. Her husband tried to cheer her up. "I'll tell you what, dear, we'll go for a drive in the foothills. Maybe we can find some Indians for you up there."

They drove to the foothills. Seeing a sign—"Native American Art Gallery"—they stopped and went in to admire the paintings. After a few minutes, the attendant walked straight up to Glenda. With no introduction, he said to her, "I've got a great-aunt. She is very old and very wise. Her name is so-and-so. She is a full-blooded Hopi Indian, and she lives in Arizona on the reservation in a little village called Second Mesa. You should go see her." He turned on his heel and walked off.

As far as I know, Glenda still hasn't visited her wise old Grandmother. It is worth mentioning, though, that Grandmother mountain mahogany is just about the only one of my plant friends who makes her home both in California and in Hopi Land.

This story shows how plant medicine connects us to the spirit of place, which is to say, the spirit of nature. The connection with nature is exhilarating and beautiful, but it is not meant to be a luxury. Connection with nature is health; health is life. Without it we shrivel and die like the artist with leukemia. With it we prosper. This is so because we are nature; we are made of dirt, rain, sunshine, minerals, and gases. How we relate to the landscape within is how we relate to the landscape without. Eating disorders and erosion of the topsoil are part of the same problem. Ecological crisis is a medical syndrome writ large. The plants already know this. They have never forgotten that the fortune of one is the fortune of all, and that is why they are generous and compassionate with humankind.

It is 1988. I have just moved to the Sierra foothills in Northern California, and I am getting to know the plant communities here. I make a dream journey to meet the spirit of the fragrant California incense cedar. She is a beautiful, brown-skinned woman who lets me know that wherever she grows, the cedar spirit is the mother of every creature who lives in the forest.

"The cedars are pleased with you," she says, "and we help you to have success with the other plant spirits. We continue to help you because of your kindness to us long ago."

"My kindness to you?" I say. "When have I ever been kind to you? Aren't we meeting now for the first time?"

"It was my cousin, the northern white cedar," she says. "Don't you recall?"

Suddenly, I do remember a scene I've forgotten for eighteen years. It is early spring in Vermont, and I am on my way to the cedar bog to cut fence posts . . .

chapter 3

SPIRIT

As I write this, my youngest child is two years old. She can barely speak, yet being with her brings me fulfillment beyond what I feel with my articulate friends. There is something special about her. In her presence I am happier, sweeter, and wiser. If you have ever loved a child, even for just a moment, you know what I mean.

That special something about my daughter is what I call *spirit*.

Do you remember those moments when you were most in touch with your own spirit? It might have happened any time: while you were looking into the eyes of a loved one, watching a beautiful sunset, facing danger, even just washing the dishes. Suddenly, you were filled with peace and energy. Life was full of deep meaning. You were, for a while, fully alive.

Chances are that when you were very young, you lived in the fullness of spirit most of the time, just as my two-year-old daughter did. If you are an adult, chances are that nowadays these experiences are rare enough to be memorable. What happened to you? Somehow your heart was broken, or you became insecure, or your self-esteem was shattered, or you were smitten by fear or anger. These terrible events, whatever they were, wounded your spirit.

If you recognize this and admit it to yourself, then you are exceptionally honest. Most of us start lying to ourselves as soon as the spirit starts to suffer. We lie to ourselves about our spiritual wounds because they hurt so much. Physical and mental pain cannot compare to the pain of losing the thing that makes life worth living. This pain is unbearable, so we cover it with anything we can, such as work, food, power, possessions, sex, romance, religion, or alcohol and drugs. The high we get from these things feeds the lie that we are okay and masks our spiritual pain. We further bolster the lie by lavishing attention on our bodies and minds.

We have all the luxuries of food, shelter, medical care, and recreation, and we can receive every conceivable form of education and therapy. But amid this affluence, no one confronts the appalling, dangerous poverty of spirit. It takes hold as we move toward adulthood. A leading cause of middle-class teenage death in the United States is suicide. Adults are not as direct as children—we choose more complicated forms of suicide. Cancer, heart disease, and drug addiction are minor concerns compared to the problem of spiritual illness. This is all the more true since these symptoms, and most others, are usually disguised forms of spiritual pain.

Technological advances in medicine have not reduced human suffering. On the contrary, wealth and technology have impoverished our spiritual life. We desperately, urgently, need medicine for the spirit, and this kind of medicine does not depend on anything money can buy, as my first encounter with the Huichol people taught me.

I have heard that in Mexico's western Sierra Madre there lives a great Huichol Indian shaman, one who was taught by a sacred plant to heal the human spirit. His name is Matsuwa, don José Ríos. It has taken me a year to locate don José and travel to his home to meet him. As I round a bend in the trail, his hamlet comes into view: children, dogs, pigs, and chickens are wandering among a handful of huts made of sticks, with thatch roofs and dirt floors.

I enter the settlement and am led to don José's hut. Here at last is the great man: a skinny, toothless, unshaven old Indian, dressed in a shabby shirt and ancient, crumbling trousers held up by a piece of twine around the waist. If this person walked by me on the street, I would not even notice him were it not for the fact that his right arm is amputated above the elbow.

Don José welcomes my companions and me. To make us feel at ease, he tells a story: "Last year an American girl came to visit. Her name was Margarita. Ay, that Margarita! She came up to me one day and said, 'Don José, I'm going to give you a massage!' I said, 'All right.' She said, 'Okay, take your clothes off!' I said, 'No!' Ay, that Margarita!"

Don José laughs. I wait for the story to continue, but that's it. Evidently this is the funniest thing that has happened all year—the old man can't stop laughing.

During the first hour of my visit, don José tells the story of Margarita six times, laughing just as hard each time. Obviously I have arrived here too late. The old man appears to be senile.

The next morning begins the ceremony don José is to lead. I have been told this is a ceremony for the young children. Since they are not yet strong enough to make a pilgrimage to the remote mountains, valleys, and springs where the gods live, the shaman will make a journey in spirit to these places, singing his adventures as he goes. Supposedly his chant will bring the souls of the children along with him so that they may be uplifted by the deities living there.

The old man takes a seat between his two assistants next to an elaborate altar. The children and their parents are sitting on the ground, rattles in hand, waiting for the spiritual voyage to begin. Don José spits out the stub of his cigarette and begins to sing in the Huichol language. The drummer picks up the rhythm, the children join in with their rattles, and the assistants chant the refrains.

All day long the children sit under the hot sun, rattling accompaniment to the shaman's song. Just yesterday they appeared to be normal, active, healthy children, and normal children do not sit still unless they are fascinated by something. I have to admit that in the cracks between my boredom and stiffness, I myself have been having colorful visions of various landscapes. I wonder what the children are seeing. Could it be that the ceremony is working, that don José is taking their spirits to meet the gods?

It is late afternoon now, and the first day of chanting will soon be over. Someone tells me that the shaman is singing about the rain god.

I notice a change in the light, and I look around. There are enormous black rainclouds over the mountains. A lightning bolt strikes a nearby peak, and thunder rolls. Within moments a rainstorm surrounds us. The village itself remains calm; the sun is still shining here. Don José sings on. After twenty minutes or so, his chant draws to a close. Everyone gets up, stretches, and strolls home. As soon as all are safe in their huts, the storm closes in and drenches the village.

The next day the children once again shake their rattles as the shaman sings from morning until evening under clear skies. Again a rainstorm suddenly appears in the surrounding mountains. As before, the storm closes in on the village only after don José concludes the ceremony and everyone is safe indoors.

A few days later, I approach don José and ask him to perform a healing on me.

"What's your problem, sonny?" he asks.

"I've got hay fever."

"What's that?"

"You know—allergies."

"Never heard of them."

"Well, sometimes my eyes get itchy and my nose runs and I sneeze a lot."

"All right, come by my house in the morning."

The next morning I present myself at his hut. He shoos away a couple of hens and welcomes me inside. He produces one of the few items of furniture in the hamlet—a low milking stool—and seats me on it. He stands in front of me, staring silently. At length he pronounces his diagnosis of the cause of my hay fever.

"You've got a girlfriend on the side, huh?"

"No, don José, I haven't been with anyone else since I've been married."

After his performance in the ceremony, I had begun to think maybe he wasn't senile after all, but now I am sure he has lost it. I have never been unfaithful to my wife.

"Nope, you've got a girlfriend on the side. Sorry, sonny, don't mean to offend you; I'm just telling you what I'm seeing . . . Hey, you are a serious case! Your pistol is about to drop off!"

With this he turns around, strides over to the wall, and reaches into a basket. He produces a small wooden wand with feathers tied to it. He approaches me and makes passes around my body with the feathers, accompanied by popping sounds made with his lips. From time to time, he puts one end of the wand on my body and places the other end to his mouth, sucking and slurping loudly. Then he makes a disgusted face and spits onto the floor a glob of what looks like thick brown mucus. He once again remarks on what a difficult case I am. He tosses the wand back into the basket and tells me to return the following day.

I notice no effect whatsoever from his treatment, but the next morning I dutifully return to his home where I am treated to the same routine as the day before. This time he seems satisfied with his work. He draws himself up to his full height and declares, "There! You're clean!" He returns the wand to the basket and then wheels around. "You're going to remember me now, sonny! You're going to remember me for the rest of your life!" He strides out of the hut.

Once again I notice no effect. I am dejected. I have come all this way for nothing. Tomorrow I start my journey back home.

When nighttime comes I can't sleep. I am lying on the ground wide awake, unable to ignore the fleas and cockroaches feasting on my body. Don José's words come to mind: "You have a girlfriend on the side." For the first time I admit to myself that in a hidden corner of my heart I never let go of the lover I had before I met my wife. That lover has been inside me, gnawing like a worm in an apple.

"Your pistol is about to drop off." An overstatement, maybe, but for sure this situation has been robbing some of my sexual energy. Well, okay, a lot of my sexual energy. How did the old guy know this?

"Now you are clean!" That is exactly how I feel! Somehow don José has sucked all the crap out of me. I feel as clear and energetic as a baby. My heart fills with love for my wife.

Two days later when I reach home, I am still full of love. My wife receives me at the door. She looks into my eyes and knows the ghost is gone.

⁓

This illiterate Indian healed my spirit and brought me to wholeness. Despite his poverty, he gave me a great treasure. Years later I found out that it is not necessary to be poor, illiterate, or Indian in order to learn deep healing from a plant; most plants will teach anyone who is interested. If you have the interest, follow up on it and see for yourself.

As a way to begin your apprenticeship with plant spirits, feel free to try the following technique. It may not turn you into as great a healer as don José—that depends on whether you are as great an apprentice as he was—but my students and I have performed many healings with the power we acquired from the following method.

Put yourself in an open and receptive state. Consider this: the mind is not subtle enough to grasp spirit or make judgments about it. How can we know what is possible? The spirit that moves through a plant might have compassion for you and take a form your mind can understand. Before you go any further, thank the plant spirits in advance for their help and hospitality. Do it aloud. This will help open you, and the spirits will like it.

Keep thankfulness in your heart as you assemble the following materials:

- A drum and someone to beat it for you (or if these are not available, use a shamanic drum recording)
- A small amount of loose tobacco
- A reliable, easy-to-use field guide on the flora of your area
- A notebook and pen (colored pencils or magic markers are also a good idea)

Go for a walk outdoors at a time and place where there are many different kinds of wild plants growing. Wander with no destination in mind. When you come across a stand of plants that are especially attractive to you, approach them. Speaking aloud, introduce yourself by name, and explain that you have come to learn from the spirit of this species. Thank the plant for summoning you and for any help it may be willing to give. Since you are asking for a gift, it is only good manners to offer one in return: sprinkle the plants with a little tobacco.

Now turn to your field guide and identify the plant to which you are speaking. (Identification is usually possible only when the plant is flowering.) Make sure the plant is not poisonous. If you have even a slight doubt about its identity, have it confirmed by a qualified botanist. There are deadly poisonous plants growing in almost every locale.

Study the plant closely. Try to memorize the shapes, colors, and geometry. Make a drawing of the plant. Observe what kind of soil it grows in, what kind of light it likes, and how it relates to insects, animals, and other plants. Smell the different parts of the plant and then, after asking its permission and forgiveness, carefully taste a tiny bit of the flowers, leaves, and root, provided they aren't poisonous.

Now that you're familiar with the plant, begin to connect with it. Be still. Take your time. Become the plant. Experience the world around you as the plant does. At this point you may be flooded with images, feelings, or information. After you return to normal consciousness, jot down your experiences in your notebook.

Return to a quiet and comfortable indoor space. You will need a monotonous, steady drumbeat of two to four cycles per second, so prepare your drummer or your audio player. (If you're using a recording, it should be approximately ten minutes in length and should have a minute or so of faster-paced drumming at the end.) Make yourself as comfortable as possible. For most people, this means lying on your back with a pillow under your neck and/or your knees. Close your eyes. Take a few deep breaths, relaxing more deeply with each one. Affirm your intention of meeting and learning from the spirit of the plant you are studying. Start the drumming.

With your eyes still closed, visualize yourself entering a hole in the earth, such as a cave, a spring, or an animal burrow. Once inside, you will find a tunnel leading downward. Go down the tunnel. Immediately, or after some time, you will see a light at the end of the tunnel; follow it. Move out of the tunnel and into the light. At this point you will have entered a different realm: the dream world. (If you don't succeed the first time, be patient. Entering the dream world takes practice.)

You may need to take a few moments to accustom yourself to the dream world. If you feel vague or distracted, remind yourself of your intention and then carry on. Once you feel confident, start looking for the plant you have come here to meet.

When you have located the plant growing in the dream world, look around. You will find a life-form associated with the plant. It might be a person, an imaginary figure, an insect, an animal, or even a light or a disembodied voice. Whatever it is, this is the form the plant spirit is taking in order to communicate with you. Approach the spirit and introduce yourself. Explain that you have come to learn, and ask if you may learn from this plant or use it in some way. If the reply is positive, then ask the spirit to teach you.

The teachings of plants come in many forms. The spirit may give you a classroom-style lecture. If so, listen intently so you can remember every detail. More often the transmission comes in nonverbal form. You may find yourself being swept into an exotic adventure. You may simply find that you experience intense emotions. In every case, the key is to remain attentive. Once you ask your question, whatever happens is part of the answer.

When you feel your dream is complete, return to the plant spirit and thank it for its help. As you take your leave, signal your drummer to give you a more rapid drumbeat. If you are using a recording, wait for the more rapid drumbeat. Quickly retrace your route: go up the tunnel, out of the hole, and return to your body. Take a few minutes of silence to mentally review what happened in your dream.

Slowly get up and record in your notebook every detail of your experience. Be complete and precise. No matter how vivid the dream, details will vanish from your memory over time unless they are written down.

Now is the time to start interpreting the dream material. Your dream may be self-explanatory, or it may require a lot of thought and contemplation. Some dreams yield their meaning only after they are illuminated by strange coincidences that take place later. This can take months or even years. Be patient.

Some time ago I was teaching a group of people in Central California to dream with the spirits in this manner. We had dreamed to meet our personal guides to the dream world, and the people in the group were sharing their experiences. One young woman, Paula, said she had met the historical Indian woman, Pocahontas, whom she called "Mother." The dream material seemed satisfying to me, but as she recounted it, Paula's tone of voice sounded disappointed, even sarcastic. I questioned her about it.

"Well," Paula said, "I grew up on a very remote farm in North Dakota. There weren't any real kids around to play with, so I played with imaginary friends. My main companion throughout my childhood was Mother Pocahontas. So, obviously, I'm just making this up, right?"

I thought that Paula's childhood relationship with the spirit of Pocahontas only made the dream more credible. I suggested that she return to Mother in her next dream and ask for some sign that their friendship was real and not just imaginary. She agreed. After the next session, Paula reported that Pocahontas had been waiting for her when she arrived. She had offered Paula a ring as a token of love. The ring would appear in ordinary reality, and then Paula would know that Mother really was her teacher. Paula was not to go looking for the ring; it would come to her.

In her dream, Paula had studied the ring closely, and afterward she recounted the stones in it, how they were cut, and the details of the setting. Also in the dream, as Paula had extended her hands to receive the gift, she noticed that her wedding ring was missing. It was precisely on the ring finger of her left hand that Mother had placed the dream ring. What, she wondered, could be the significance of this? The entire experience was curious to her, but not entirely convincing.

Some time after this class was over, I moved to Northern California. A year went by. I forgot about Paula and Pocahontas. Then one day I got a letter. Paula wanted to let me know what had happened since the class:

Only a couple of months after you were here, I was walking by a jewelry store in San Luis Obispo, and I saw a ring that was very similar to the one Mother gave me in my dream. I got real excited and was just about to go in and buy it, but I realized that the ring wasn't exactly the same. Anyway, she had told me not to go looking for it, that it would come to me, so I passed it by. The next strange thing happened only two weeks ago—I lost my wedding ring! I still can't explain how it happened. I never took that ring off, not to do the dishes or shower or anything. I just looked at my hand one day, and it wasn't there! I was so upset. Michael and the kids and I scoured the house and the car. I retraced my steps to the Safeway. I even went so far as to rent a metal detector and go over every inch of the yard, but no good—it was gone!

After that, just last week, I got a letter from my old friend Karen in Tucson. I hadn't heard from her in about seven years. Anyway, in the letter Karen said that she still thinks about me a lot. In fact, just a few days before she was walking past a jewelry store, and she saw a ring in the window. She just knew that it was mine, so she went in and bought it for me. There was this little package in the letter. I opened it up, and it was *the ring!* Exactly, down to the tiniest detail! I was amazed! I had to try it on immediately . . . There was only one finger that it fit: the ring finger on my left hand!

I thought you would enjoy hearing about this. I guess I've changed my mind about Mother. Thanks a lot for the workshop.

In addition to dreaming and accepting the wisdom of sacred plant teachers, there is a third way to learn how to heal the spirit: the way of pilgrimage. There are special places in the world that would appear to be ordinary geographical forms—mountains, caves, springs, groves—but in reality they are god-forms, endowed with sacred doorways through which a pilgrim can gain special knowledge and capacity. Many such places exist; they are well known to local indigenous peoples throughout the world.

Pilgrimage is one of the most powerful ways of receiving spirit medicine. It is also one of the most dangerous, for great power always must be engaged impeccably, lest harm be done. An everyday activity like driving a car provides an example of the care needed to handle power. Many people take for granted the power in the hands of the driver, without considering that to arrive safely at his or her destination, the driver must know how to control the vehicle and understand and comply with traffic rules. If we do not drive on the correct side of the road, for instance, death or dismemberment is sure to follow.

Just as we need a qualified driving instructor to teach us how to drive a car, we need a competent, properly initiated guide to show us how to make pilgrimages. The "rules of the road" for each site are not negotiable; they are part of the place itself. Knowledge of the rules is passed down from generation to generation. My teacher, don Guadalupe González Ríos, received much of his medicine from pilgrimages to the Wind Tree. Don Lupe, as I called him, received his instruction from his uncle, who was known as a great shaman. The uncle had been guided, in turn, by his own elder. The Huichol lineage has remained intact since the beginnings of humanity, but in other places knowledge is lost and difficult to restore.

Anyone who can pass the exam can get a driver's license, but to get a "pilgrim's license" you need commitment, endurance, and an invitation from the site you wish to visit. The invitation is delivered by the ancestors, who see if you are related to the land and its people. Without an invitation, you'll be considered an interloper, and sacred sites have big, burly bouncers to deal with interlopers. You really are not interested in the kind of bouncing they do!

There are also human guardians: the indigenous peoples to whom the sites were given as part of their homelands. Invaders of European descent have taken so much that did not belong to them—game, timber, waters, fish, minerals, the land itself, even the lives of the people. In their grief and anger, many indigenes say, "It's never enough for these whites! Now they want to take our sacred traditions too!" They are not eager to share the all-important protocols for approaching sacred places. The wisest, having resolved their rage, still know that a visitor must be invited by the site itself. When the door is closed to the visitor, it is open to mischief.

Due to some novel conditions we will discuss in chapter 6, there are genetically European people who nevertheless have soul relatedness to lands and peoples elsewhere. When they demonstrate exceptional respect, patience, and courage, they can sometimes become traditional pilgrims at places exotic to their birth and immediate blood ancestry.

Of course, there are also millions of European peoples still living in their own homelands. Access to pilgrimage sites in Europe presents a different obstacle: lineages of tradition-holders have long since been broken, so no one knows the protocols anymore. Efforts have been made to retrieve the sacred knowledge, but they have been at best incomplete and contaminated with wishful thinking and modern "new age" assumptions. The good news, though, is that as of this writing there are some authentic projects working to revive the traditions and reawaken the places of pilgrimage. This can be done only with extraordinary divine intervention, but there have been many times in the past when people lost their sacred teachings and practices; when conditions in society ripen, the Divine always finds a way to restore what has been lost.

Despite the pitfalls (or maybe because of them), pilgrimage offers blessed opportunities for humankind. The sacred sites can transform the pilgrim and make him or her capable of receiving and holding medicine of the spirit.

chapter 4

MEDICINE
AND DREAMS

Recall one of your most vivid nighttime dreams and how real it felt. Dreams have all the characteristics of waking experience: convincing sights, smells, sound, touch; powerful emotional content; and the ability to create effects in the "real" world. It is not uncommon for men to ejaculate while asleep, for example, and people have been known to die of heart attacks during traumatic dreams. There may be different rules in particular dreams; you might be able to fly or perform other unusual feats, for example. Nevertheless, the dream world has a consistent structure, just as the waking world does. The differences between the dream and waking worlds are difficult to pinpoint, yet we generally feel that dream objects are "made up," while in daily life we accept "real" objects made of "solid matter." There is a story of a wealthy and powerful king in ancient India that illustrates this point.

One day the king of the land was reclining on his favorite couch and being fanned by slaves, while a handmaiden massaged his feet. He had just eaten a meal of the finest delicacies, and despite the spectacle of musicians and beautiful dancing girls before him, he became drowsy and fell asleep.

In his slumber, the king dreamed he was a miserable beggar wandering along a country road. He had not eaten for several days, and when he came across a mango tree laden with ripe fruit, he could not resist the temptation. Just as he was stuffing mangoes into his bag, the farmer appeared with a stick in his hand and gave the beggar a ferocious beating. The sting of the stick on his back made the beggar cry out in pain, and the noise of his own pitiful cries awoke him. Once again he was the great king in his palace being pampered with every luxury.

The king was soon comforted by his attendants and fell asleep once more. Again he assumed the identity of the hungry beggar; again he picked the mangoes; again he knew the farmer's stick; again he cried out in pain and woke to his courtly life. This time the king was very upset. It was quite some time before he managed to fall asleep, but when he did, it was only to relive the painful experience for a third time.

When he awoke this time, the king was beyond consolation. "Who am I really?" he called out, "A beggar, or a king? Which of these two worlds is the real one?"

None of the courtiers dared hazard an answer to the question. In frustration, the king declared that all the philosophers of his kingdom should appear before him. Whoever could answer his question would be richly rewarded, but he who should fail would be cast into prison.

Most of the intelligentsia of that land were soon wasting away in the royal dungeon, but finally a wise one resolved the king's question. He was a young boy who had been an object of scorn due to his grotesque appearance. His response to the king was that neither the dream nor the waking experience was real.

Modern science makes the same point in a less poetic way. Research reveals matter to be empty space with a few tiny particles in it. The particles are energy phenomena. There is no "stuff" in the universe; it is all made out of energy.

As quantum physics explores the nature of energy, some fascinating qualities come to light. For example, in observing a "particle," it is impossible to determine both its momentum and its location at the same time, because the very act of observing a characteristic causes it to leap out of the probable state and become actual. All other characteristics are still merely probabilities at that moment. To put this another way, energy has certain tendencies. The moment we look for one of those tendencies, it manifests itself, while all other tendencies remain latent. This is a bit like getting to know a person. If you provoke someone's anger, their tendency to express affection cannot be observed at the same time. One might say that energy knows when it is being watched, and it behaves to fulfill our expectations. Energy responds to us. It is conscious.

According to modern physics, although our world appears real and solid, it is actually an insubstantial realm whose features shift according to the psyche of the person who is observing it. The first paragraph of this chapter described dream worlds the same way. Thus, the young sage's explanation to the monarch was truth: the palace splendors and the farmer's stick were both illusions—made of the same "stuff." Many forms of shamanic healing use the timelessness and porousness of dreams to enable shamans to make their diagnosis. Modern science and ancient wisdom concur, then, in describing our world as a dream—a tissue of appearances made of energy and consciousness.

The dream of waking life appears to be longer lived, or at least more repetitive than our nighttime dreams. In actuality, though, all dreams are timeless. When I was an anthropology student, I read the account of an ethnographer who had spent considerable time among Australian aborigines. He had heard stories of the tracking skills of one particular hunter; the stories were so incredible that he was certain they were fraudulent. When he finally met the tracker, he challenged him to follow the trail of a long trek he had made with another aborigine years before. He was certain this was impossible and that no trail could remain for such a long time. The tracker was happy to take up the challenge, though, and the moment he was shown the starting point, he took off at a trot and ran the whole course of the journey without even pausing to examine the spoor. The anthropologist was humbled and apologetic. He asked the aborigine how he had accomplished this feat. "It was easy," the tracker replied. "I just went back to the time you made the journey, and I ran alongside you."

These anecdotes serve to illustrate that dreams—including the dream of waking life—exist outside the flow of time.

Another interesting characteristic of dreams is that they are permeable and overlapping. One dream interpenetrates another, and a dreamer can move freely among his own dreams and those of others. A woman with three daughters recently told me that she shared a dream with two of her daughters one night. The dream accurately foretold a mysterious, life-threatening illness that befell the third daughter in India.

One of the games I like to play with my students goes like this: one member of the class describes a favorite location in the dream world. That student then enters his or her dream, goes to the described location, and prepares some surprises for the others. A few minutes later the others also enter dream reality, find the first student, and discover the surprises waiting for them. Then everyone returns to ordinary reality. The first student writes down on a piece of paper an account of the surprises he or she prepared. The paper is folded and kept from view as each person describes his or her experience. After all the stories have been told, the first student unfolds the paper and reads the initial account. The object of the game is to demonstrate that we can enter someone else's dream. Invariably, some students get all the surprises right, most get a few of them, and everybody gets at least one.

I am convinced that the universe is a very complicated dream. In order to create it and keep it going, God the Dreamer dreams a multitude of lesser dreamers. Each of these lesser dreamers, or gods, is in charge of dreaming up one part of the world. For example, the stone god has a long dream that brings the stones into being, and when the rain god dreams of showers, the rains fall. Their dreams overlap, and the stones get wet.

Human beings are like gods—we ourselves are dreamers. As time goes on, we live more and more within our own dreams and less and less within the dream of nature. This is hard to see. The fish does not see the water, and the Los Angeleno does not see the smog. Nevertheless, it is very important that we come to know the difference between the human dream and the dream of nature, or else we will never understand medicine.

One of the foundations of modern life is the dream of time as a mechanical procession of discreet, uniform units. In this dream, seconds click by in single file from an unknowable future through a fleeting present into the jaws of an irretrievable past. Virtually all humankind has agreed on this view, making possible a regimentation of human effort that was unthinkable before hours, minutes, and seconds were dreamed up. Clock time makes factories possible.

By contrast, Australian aborigines traditionally live not by clock time, but by what is called the dreamtime. The dreamtime is a timeless realm in which the Ancestors sing into existence every feature of the natural world. For those who live by the dreamtime, the world is sacred and inviolable. Not a single pebble must be disturbed from its place. The people of the dreamtime will never produce a laptop computer, but they will never produce ecological crisis either.

The Western dream of time is dualistic in that it divides the web of existence into two irreconcilable parts: the present, which is real, and the nonpresent, which is not real. According to this scheme, the aboriginal tracker's feat is impossible and absurd because an event cannot occur simultaneously in the past and the present. I give thanks to that Australian and his anthropologist friend for gently suggesting where the absurdity truly lies.

Dualism is the proto-dream underlying clock time and all modern dreaming. Dualism might be defined as the illusion that there are two discreet principles in the universe: self and other. Dualism implies isolation, conflict, and a continuous struggle of opposing forces. For this reason, actions based on dualistic vision are simplistic, aggressive, and destructive.

For example, a farmer dreams that his livestock is part of "self" and predators are "other." Immediately there is conflict, and the conflict suggests a simple, aggressive solution: destroy the predators. This is precisely the solution humanity has adopted over the past few thousand years. Since dualism is blind to complexity, we have failed to notice that in destroying predators we have disrupted the ecosystem in such a way as to impoverish productive lands and turn them into deserts.[1] The dualistic dream engenders an endless procession of conflict, aggression, and destruction as each "solution" creates new problems to be attacked. One who lives in the dream of dualism lives in a battlefield, as a walk through any city will attest.

In the Dreamer's dream of nature there is no duality, no separation into self and other, no conflict, aggression, or destruction. In the dream of nature, when a predator kills and eats an animal, it is not "us" against "them." In nature, all are "us." A slow, sick, or injured animal is provided to predators for the benefit of all. The health of the herd is maintained as the predator feeds its family. The dream of nature is a complex web of mutuality in which each part supports the other.

This is the most important difference between the dream of man and the dream of nature: nature dreams of unity and bliss, while man dreams of isolation and violence. Humans need unity and bliss to maintain their health of spirit. The dualistic dream starves the spirit and gives rise to the gamut of illnesses of body and soul. The job of medicine, then, is to nourish the spirit by bringing people into the source of wellbeing—the dream of nature.

Nature is dreamed by the gods. The gods are dreamed by God. To commune with nature is to commune with the Divine, so healing is truly a religious rite with healer as priest.

Let's say a patient consults me with a concern about a respiratory infection. I do not try to kill microorganisms in her lungs. In fact, I ignore her symptoms entirely, because I know there is no "them" to fight against. It's all "us" trying to work through something for the benefit of this woman.

So what is trying to be worked through here? I speak with the woman and find she has stifled her grief over the death of her sister. What should have been discharged through weeping has lodged in her lungs and made her susceptible to infection. Why has she stifled her grief? She suffers under the illusion that she is weak and worthless. She secretly fears that if she allowed her grief to surface, she would dissolve in the tide of her tears.

Just as the stones are dreamed into existence by the stone god and the rain by the rain god, so each plant is dreamed into being by the god or spirit of the species. I have entered the dreams of many plants, and now I select one who dreams of inner strength. I ask the spirit of this plant to include my patient in its dreaming. Immediately the woman notices a feeling of peace, accompanied by ineffable sadness. Without knowing why, she bursts into tears.

By the time she reaches home after our appointment, she is weeping uncontrollably. This continues for two days, interrupted only by spasms of coughing that produce thick, old mucus. By the time the weeping stops, her respiratory infection has cleared. More important, she now enters a rich new experience of herself and her life.

Several years ago my left shoulder joint suddenly froze and became painful. There was no apparent cause for this affliction, and each of the healers I consulted failed to affect it. One evening it occurred to me to ask one of my plant spirit allies for help with this condition. The spirit's response was to tell me I had to move out of Santa Barbara. I loved Santa Barbara. I had made my home there for many years, and I was not eager to leave. At the very least I wanted an explanation. I argued with the plant to no avail. At length I relented and assured it I would move. Instantly my shoulder got 50 percent better. That gave me the conviction I needed to uproot my family and start a new life in an unfamiliar place.

It took about a year to accomplish the move. Just after we arrived in Northern California, my father came down with a terminal illness. Because I now lived relatively close to him, I was able to attend to him, heal our strained relationship, and be with him at the moment of his death. In addition, after we left Santa Barbara a ferocious fire, whipped by eighty-mile-per-hour winds, swept through the canyon where we had lived, destroying our former home and seven hundred other houses. One person lost her life in that blaze. Her remains were found in the creek bed beside the ruins of our house. When I moved north, my shoulder was completely healed, but that was incidental.

Frozen shoulder, lung infection, whatever the complaint is, it's always the same thing: something beneficial trying to happen. There is no conflict, no enemy, no disease—only the opportunity to bring someone out of the dream of strife into the dream of wholeness.

There are many medicines to help a person enter the dream of wholeness. Although plants are well suited to the task, it is not necessary to use them. Two things are necessary, however. First, the medicine must be nondualistic. Second, the medicine must have the power of dreams. A practitioner does not acquire this power by accident. Lofty, well-focused intention is required, and intention must be married to knowledge and skill.

The dream world is not limited by time or space, and plants in particular access the source of healing, the divine dream of nature. To arrive at this understanding, in this book's first section we have examined the four components of plant spirit medicine dreams—namely plants, spirit, medicine, and dreams. Along the way, we have considered shamanism; pilgrimage; Native American and Native Australian philosophies; and the nature of humans, time, and reality. We have seen the goal of this form of healing and have understood there is a method to help reach that goal.

After all this, we can finally answer the question "Am I making this up?" with a resounding "yes and no." No, I am not making up what the plant spirits give me or what they do for my patients, and yes, I am making up most of the rest of my life.

chapter 5

VIEW

I was sitting around a fire one night, talking with a number of people, when a man I had never met shared this story: One day he had been sitting in an armchair in his back yard, studying an ancient scripture. Suddenly he remembered an urgent errand, so he set the fragile book on the chair and drove to town to attend his business.

While the man was in town, black clouds blew in without warning. He knew rain would soon follow, and he feared for the fate of the scripture. At that moment, he recalled my book and the story of how I came to relate to rain as a living presence. As the storm was now upon him, he prayed to the rain, explaining the preciousness of his book and asking that it be spared from destruction. He arrived home to find the cloudburst had soaked *everything* in the yard—except the armchair and the scripture, which were dry.

This man was well steeped in the Western, dualistic view of the world. The story in my book, though, resonated in him, and he was open to the resonance. It was as if he said to himself, "What Eliot discovered feels right somehow. Maybe the world is *not* mechanical and distant. Maybe it hears me and responds. Never mind if it seems silly or embarrassing; I'm going to speak to the rain. I will explain my concern, make my request, and see what happens." What happened was this: the unity view proved itself correct.

Had this man approached the situation from the dualistic view, that would also have proved itself correct, for the premise of dualism is eternal conflict between *self* (the man and his book) and *other* (the rain), in which the *other* is always the problem to be destroyed or overpowered. Dualism has yet to discover how to overpower or destroy rain on short notice, so the dualistic view would have only this to offer: "See, I told you so; the world is your enemy."

Here is another example of the effect of view: When I had my first interview with the spirit of a plant, fifteen or so other Western people were also talking to plants about healing and knowledge. What came out of my interview was the rediscovery of an ancient medicine and the development of a way to reintroduce it to the Western world. What came out of their interviews, so far as I know, was simply an interesting conversation. I had an advantage the others did not have: I was speaking from a traditional, nondualistic view of healing. It was not a theoretical view; I had lived and worked in it successfully for ten years. Naturally, the plant world spoke back to me in my own language, accepting and expanding my view.

What was it in the man with the scripture that resonated with the nondual view I wrote about? What was it in me that resonated with the Chinese Five-Element view of Fire, Earth, Metal, Water, and Wood? If there had been nothing in us to resonate with, he would not have prayed, and I would not have done the work I did. His manuscript would have been ruined, and he would still see the world as his adversary. My conversation with a plant spirit would have borne poor fruit, and I would similarly be at odds with the world. I say what resonated in us was a natural, innate nondualistic view.

Since both traditional wisdom and modern science agree that the world shows up according to how we view it, it is worthwhile considering what "view" is. First, some words about what view is *not*. It is not a set of opinions to agree or disagree with. It is not a belief system. It cannot be acquired by studying or reading books. View is not something we can think our way into. We have it in our bones. We live in it. Usually it is as transparent as water is to fish.

Yes, the world shows up according to how we view it, but this does not mean we can get the world to produce what we want by changing our thoughts. Trying to get the world to produce what we want is itself a product of the dualistic view that sees the world as an *other* to be controlled or exploited. View is not the same as our thoughts; it is more like the seedbed of our thinking.

Education today claims to be about passing on information, but in fact, it is more about getting the young to take on the dualistic view. By force of law, children are put into situations that reward competition and individual achievement. Demonstrations of cooperation and empathy are discouraged or even punished. Over and over, the young have these experiences drilled into them. In time, "me against the world" seeps into their bones until it becomes "truth." "Life is about getting what you want, and you don't have to consider the cost to your enemy": this is how the world works for most people today, because most people see it that way. Almost nobody realizes that this "truth" is nothing more than the product of their view. In fact, few people realize they have a view at all.

The Western view produces results that are useful in some ways. When I am driving a car, for example, the modern Western view of time and space serves me well. When I am doing healing work, though, the traditional Chinese view and the traditional Huichol view produce results unobtainable in more conventional ways. Plant spirit medicine healers and Huichol shamans routinely do things that are flat-out impossible by Western standards, but this does not bother us. The results speak for themselves. They are simply expressions of how the world works from our points of view.

I know a conventional physician whose daughter was born with several serious health conditions. I offered to set up an appointment for the child with my teacher, the Huichol shaman don Guadalupe. The treatment would be totally noninvasive, I explained. The girl would just be lightly brushed with feathers. The doctor's mother offered to pay for the treatment. He was reluctant at first, but he finally agreed to have his child seen. The day before the appointment, he rang me to say he was cancelling "because my wife and I don't believe in this sort of thing." The child died some time later.

Of course, there is no way of knowing what would have happened had the child been treated. My point is that invalidating other views denies us access to their possible benefits. The Western view is not the only one; there are many. Each view is valid and offers unique capabilities. Insisting on one's own view as the only truth reveals deep insecurity on the part of the speaker. In extreme cases, that insecurity can cause the holders of the "truth" to exterminate the holders of other views. Many indigenous peoples have died this way, and the extermination efforts go on to this day.

So back to the question: What *is* view?

We need certain equipment—arms, legs, mouth, and so on—to get along in the world. We don't create this equipment ourselves; we don't acquire it in school. We inherit it from our ancestors. We must also be spiritually equipped; we need a view for seeing and relating and acting in the world. Like our body, our view is also inherited from our ancestors. It is as much a part of us as our temperament or the color of our hair. It is part of our soul.

Just as there are many different peoples brought forth from different lands, there are many ancestral views, each with its unique possibilities and limitations. What they have in common is this: they are all nondualistic. In the case of the man with the scripture, his ancestral soul view resonated with my story about the rain god. My soul view resonated with the Chinese Five Elements and later recognized itself in the Huichol view.

What of the modern dualistic view? It has brought forth a society that is unsustainable. It cannot be an ancestral view, for if the ancestors' lives had not been sustained, we would not be here today. No doubt people have always had some tendency to dualism, but it was a problem to deal with rather than a view to live out of. Those societies that invest in it too heavily collapse because dualism does not support life.

The modern view alienates us from our innate connectedness. It is a conditioned view, not a natural one. This is good news, because the nature of a person will always be their nature, and whatever is conditioned can be deconditioned.

Those who become students of plant spirit medicine find that the accumulation of information is important, but secondary. The main work is to break down assumptions about how the world works, while at the same time nourishing and reinforcing the reawakened ancestral soul view.

Deep down, no one really wants the alienated view this society insists on. The soul wants to express itself with its own limbs and its own voice. It wants to see with its own eyes, to hear with its own ears. It wants to invoke the magically connected world to which it belongs. Only in this way do we come to know ourselves and be in good relationship with the beings, both human and nonhuman, around us. To be alienated produces much illness, much suffering, and a longing for what plant spirits can provide: the feeling of being at home in the world.

Fred was a friendly, good-natured farmer who had taken on the modern view with zest. I was surprised he consulted me, but I reminded myself that illness can open us in unexpected ways. In any case, he certainly needed help beyond what conventional medicine had provided. His breathing was so labored that the smallest effort had become a mountainous challenge. I treated Fred three times; after each session, he happily reported more tasks he was once again able to perform. In order to hold onto his gains and continue to progress, I explained, he would need to do a bit of homework. "The homework might seem odd," I said, "but why not try it and see whether it works. If it doesn't, you will have lost nothing but a bit of time. If it does, you will have gained a lot. "

Now I had to speak to Fred from an unconventional view, but since my treatment had brought good results so far, I figured there was a good chance I could get through to him. "I don't know if you've thought about this," I said, "but some people say the land itself and the creatures that live on it have feelings and would like to have some say about what happens to their home. Do you think that could possibly be true?"

"I dunno," Fred answered. "I suppose there could be something to it."

"Well, to me it makes a lot of sense," I said. "You know, I've asked myself why you haven't found help with your health before now, and I think it has something to do with that."

"What do you mean?"

"Well," I answered, "I think it has to do with the pond."

"The pond?"

"Yes. When the stream on your farm was bulldozed to create the dam that formed the pond, it seems the stream got sore about not being asked how it felt about the matter. It would like a little apology and some peace offerings. Kind of like bringing your wife flowers after you've had a tiff. Do you think you might be willing to do that?"

"What would I have to do, exactly?" Fred asked.

I outlined some seasonal visits and the appropriate gifts to be left at the stream.

"I couldn't walk all the way down there—not in the state I'm in," Fred objected.

"Your son could drive you down there on the tractor," I replied. "Like I said, why not give it a try? You've got nothing to lose and everything to gain."

"You think that could help my breathing?"

"If I didn't think so, I wouldn't be saying this."

"All right, I'll give it a go!"

But Fred did not give it a go. Nine months later he had not visited the stream, his symptoms had returned, and he had forgotten or denied he had received any help at all. Even a skeptical experiment in ancestral view was too big a leap for him to consider.

Donald was a much younger man who was crippled not by shortness of breath but by mysterious pain and stiffness in his legs, hips, and low back. He had been strong and athletic before the onset of his condition. Like Fred, he had not been helped with conventional care. Also like Fred, he had got himself in trouble with the waters.

Donald had made a modest investment in a hot springs resort. This seemed innocuous enough at first, but I noticed that the young man's health problems began shortly afterward. Looking at the situation through ancestral view, I saw there was indeed a relationship. The spring was a sacred site that was unhappy about its commercial development as a resort. It had blessings to offer, and it did not want them dishonored or ignored. Like Fred's illness—like all illness—the young man's pain was a call to awareness, an invitation to relationship and resolution.

Another sacred spring of my acquaintance offered to broker an arrangement for Donald. He was to undertake a traditional pilgrimage to the second spring and leave prayers and sacred offerings there. If all went well, the first spring would accept this as a gift honoring all springs, and Donald would be on good terms all around. The pilgrimage, though, required rigorous preparation, long and dangerous travel, and considerable expense.

I felt the expense might be a deal-breaker, because Donald was a man of small means. I made the offer anyway, and after thinking it over for several weeks, he accepted. The preparation was done, the expenses paid, the offerings placed. Within a few days after the trip was completed, his pain was gone.

Donald, like Fred, was presented with the proposition that springs are alive, aware, and related to us. Even though it challenged his "common sense," Donald risked acting from the ancestral view, and the world responded in kind.

chapter 6

ANCESTORS

When I was beginning to work with plant spirit medicine, I hadn't found any elders to guide me. I had questions about that: Did no one know about plant spirit medicine because I was inventing something new? (That seemed unlikely.) Was I delusional? (No, my patients were getting good results.) So where was the medicine coming from? Who was supporting it? Slowly I began to discover some of its unseen yet important sponsors: the Ancestors.

As we saw in chapter 5, all people have in our soul an ancestral view of the world. This view is passed down to us from our forebears, just as our genes are. While ancestral soul views differ from one people to the next, all have this in common: they see everything as alive, aware, and related. When a traditional indigenous person looks at a plant, he does not see an object. He sees a spirit expressing itself through its form, lifecycles, and interaction with everything around it. When he uses the plant for healing, he knows he is calling upon a spirit being. In the eyes of the ancestors, all plant medicine is plant spirit medicine.

Years ago I read an article about the Kashaya Pomo Indian healer and ceremonial leader Lorin Smith. As a young man in California, he found partying more interesting than his ancestral ways, but to his surprise, he began to be instructed in his dreams by Tom Smith, a long-dead relative who had been a respected medicine man. Guided by an ancestor he had never met, Lorin himself became a shaman and reintroduced his people to many of their traditions. This story seemed to suggest the ancestors are not simply gone when they die. Apparently they could be still around, with help and guidance to offer the living.

Eventually I went to a ceremony presided over by Lorin. I arrived early at his roundhouse, and he introduced me to a friendly middle-aged man who knew more than a thousand traditional songs. We struck up a conversation. The song keeper worked as a janitor in a nearby high school. What sort of work did I do?

At this point, I had not met anyone who had heard of the kind of work I did. I did not want this impressive traditionalist to think I was a starry-eyed flake. At the same time, I wasn't there to hide anything.

"I do plant spirit medicine, and I teach others about it," I said.

"Yeah," he replied, "that's good work." Apparently he considered this completely normal.

"Do you know any plant songs?" I asked.

"Sure, lots. Let's see . . . there are a lot of bay tree songs. The bay is sacred to us; we use it in our ceremonies and healings. Madrone too. But I can't sing those songs right now; they are for certain occasions, you know."

In this man's reluctance to sing the sacred songs out of context, I felt the beautiful relationship Pomo people have with the plant spirits of their land. Somehow I knew those relationships were built and nurtured by many generations of ancestors. I felt the presence of those ancestors, still looking over the people, helping preserve the ways that had given the ancient ones fruitful lives.

In the roundhouse I began to discover who is supporting plant spirit medicine: the Ancestors of every people honor plant spirits for their gifts of healing. When I approached the spirits respectfully, the Ancestors were interested in helping me. When they saw I was willing to share the medicine with others, they became even more interested. In fact, they help all who practice plant spirit medicine. It seems they consider the practice an important benefit, worthy of their support.

Humans and plants have lived together for a long time. When I say a long time, I mean longer than the last few hundreds or thousands of years of neglect and dishonor. Ancestral relationships with plants are still present in the land as a field of potential. Whether he knows it or not, a plant spirit medicine healer brings his patient into that field. The healer has a personal relationship with plants, but that in itself does not deliver the full effect. Personal relationship is meant to open a doorway to the ancestral field, which has greater capacity than any individual. I discovered this while working with Joe Pye weed.

Joe Pye weed is a prominent plant of wet, marshy places throughout most of the eastern and central United States. Some say Joe Pye was a Native American healer famous for curing the gamut of ailments with this single herb. Attracted by its lore and beauty, I introduced myself to the plant, offered tobacco, and asked about its medicine. I understood it to say it had something to do with the element of fire, but the dream was vague and unsatisfying, so I did not call on it for years. Just as I had come to know rain as a god, later on, other natural forces also revealed themselves as gods. Fire had become my primary tutor, and it was the God of Fire who cleared up my confusion and connected my Joe Pye dream to the ancestral field.

It seems that among many peoples the sacred name of the God of Fire was treated with such respect that it would only be uttered under special ceremonial circumstances, as if one could pronounce the name only a certain number of times in one's life. When someone wanted to refer to this deity, he substituted the name of a shaman known to have fire medicine. Joe Pye was such a shaman. "Joe Pye" was a circumspect way of saying "fire."

Fire brings us into relationship, and in relationships messages are exchanged. We send them to each other by messenger services like our gestures (nods, frowns, waving hello or goodbye) and our spoken words ("The doors open at nine o'clock," "Please pass the bananas," "I love you"). Our tone of voice also conveys many messages; said in a certain tone, "I love you" can really mean, "I'm angry with you." Text, whether on the page or the screen, is the driest messenger of all.

In the world of plant spirit medicine, Joe Pye weed is a messenger service. It works like this:

From: Healer
To: Plant spirit I am in relationship with
Via: Joe Pye weed
Message: Please come now. Help this person.
With gratitude and love, Healer

Perhaps the historical Joe Pye *did* heal many afflictions with what seemed to be a single plant.

I had already been using a plant messenger to summon the spirits, and I thought this was an innovation. But I found out it was no such thing. The messenger function was already in the field of possibilities, thanks to agreements made between ancestors and plants long before.

I called on Lorin Smith again several years after our meeting in his roundhouse. I was still learning about the Ancestors; this time the learning was about the fierceness of their grace.

A young woman I'll call Renee consulted me. She explained that her mother had been afflicted with an illness beginning with pains and paralysis of the legs and hips. All sorts of specialists had been consulted, but they provided neither explanation nor cure. The illness had progressed slowly; eventually it had taken her life.

For several months, Renee had been experiencing the same mysterious symptoms. Again, doctors had not been helpful. Was she doomed to the same fate as her mother? I did my best to look at the situation with ancestral eyes, and I saw that the house where Renee was living—the same house where her mother had lived and died—had been built on top of a native burial ground. The ancestors saw this as disrespectful and dangerous, so they sent the mother messages to correct the offense. As each message went unheard, the next became stronger, until finally they realized: she had been deafened by her culture. She would never be able to hear the ancestors until they brought her to their realm. In the afterlife she would be taught to honor them. She would carry her learning into the next lifetime. She would teach her future children what she had learned, and her children would teach their children so that generations to come would listen to the ancestors for the wisdom needed to live well with the land.

In this life, if there were to be a cure for Renee, I was sure she would have to demonstrate due respect. Since her house was in original Pomo territory, I asked her to contact Lorin, tell him my diagnosis, and ask if he could suggest some offerings to send the right message to his ancestors. Lorin visited her home and concurred with my view. He prescribed a series of offerings to be made at each season of the year. Most of the offerings were plant substances.

Renee contacted me three years later. She had made the offerings, left the house, and moved on with her life. Her health was fine.

chapter 7

EMOTION

Here are three popular movie themes:

1. It's the big championship game, and our team is behind by a single point. There is only *one minute* left to play!

2. She is totally gorgeous and a really good person. He is sexy too, but so *clueless* about women! They have a romantic fling, and she falls for him. But soon she is wounded by his male ego and ends the affair. She packs her bags and buys a ticket to a distant country where she can start a new life without him. Now he realizes he loves and needs her. Can he grow up and win her back before it's too late?

3. The enemy has a powerful secret weapon. Led by Thane the Brave, our raiders sneak into the enemy fortress and make off with the devilish device. Now they are looking for a way out of the inner chamber. Thane sneezes. A dog barks. The guards send up the alarm. If our men get caught, all is lost!

The excitement of the movies is in the chase. Whether the characters are chasing a sports championship, romance, or the triumph over evil, a good chase scene is nerve-wracking and exciting. Fear can be fun!

At the movies you can also have fun getting angry with the bad guys. And if the good guys win, you get a flush of happiness. When the good guys lose, you get deliciously sad or sympathetic. You go to the movies to taste emotions—fear, anger, happiness, sadness, sympathy, grief.[2] Even when you just talk about good movies, the emotion of them makes you glow, because to feel emotion is to feel *alive*.

Life calls you to respond to every situation, and to answer the call, an emotion arrives, opens a doorway, and pushes you into a landscape of possibilities of response. For example, in the face of fire in your office building, fear might lead you to grab the fire extinguisher, pull the fire alarm, exit the building, drop and roll, or even freeze in panic.

At the same time, there are things you cannot do in the landscape of fear: Let's say you are a man on a camping trip with your wife. It is a warm, moonlit night. No one else is around, and the two of you are happily making love. Suddenly a mother grizzly bear appears with her cubs. She stands up threateningly on her hind legs. Now she lowers herself. Growling and baring her teeth, she starts ripping your tent apart with her claws. Fear closes a door to happiness; you lose your erection. The door to self-preservation now opens.

Even in the least dramatic situations, emotion is always present, closing and opening doors and pushing us to respond to the world. In fact, there are no doors to action other than the emotional ones. Everything you do is motivated by feeling.

If that is true, then why do we spend so much time and money watching movies that stir our feelings? Furthermore, aren't some of our actions motivated by reason and logic rather than emotional urges? And how can emotion be present when we feel blank? The answers to these questions have to do with fear.

Fear has a healthy protective function: in the face of danger (angry grizzly clawing into your tent), fear gives you what you need in order to overpower the threat (shoot the bear) or run away from it. At the same time, people these days live with chronic stress, anxiety, concern, and even panic, without being in clear and present danger. This unhealthy, unproductive fear is generated by the mind, also sometimes called the ego.

The mind itself is an elaboration of fear. In our society, which idol-izes the intellect, this might seem a preposterous claim, but consider this: we humans cannot take care of our survival as other animals do—with beak, wing, fang, or claw. We have special equipment of our own, though. Unlike other animals, we rely on the creativity and adaptability of our minds to come up with strategies for feeding and protecting ourselves. Everything from sharpening a stick to the elaborate infrastructures of a modern city is a product of our minds' concern with avoiding the loss of life or any other seeming loss. The emotional energy that produces concern for survival is fear. It is not coincidental that the ancient Chinese sages recognized that the element of Water, which expresses itself as the emotion of fear, gives rise to what they called "cleverness," or what we might call "intelligence."

For all its cleverness, the mind has a one-track agenda: to protect you from the possibility of loss. Of course, this agenda is doomed to failure. Loss is unavoidable. You, like everyone, will lose loved ones, opportunities, and eventually your own life. Besides, there is more to life than just loss; there is love and laughter, sympathy and anger, and all manner of rich experiences. But this obvious truth does not deter the mind. It sees an invading bear in every situation, and it applies the only remedy fear can provide: fight or flight. It fights to control the nonexistent grizzly with any weapon it can get, in the name of avoiding loss.

Ours is a society that feels justified in killing tens of thousands of men, women, and children to protect themselves from imaginary grizzly bears such as nonexistent weapons of mass destruction. That society grew from people who arrived on new shores and saw in the primeval forests, rich soils, abundant wildlife, and clean waters only the necessity of getting the original human inhabitants out of the way and producing material gain for themselves. Today, we are a society that creates and maintains extrava-gant infrastructures to protect ourselves from the very natural world that supports us—without considering how much it costs the environment or our descendants. This society is deeply invested in the fearful view of the mind. And it is dangerously out of balance.

On the individual level, the mind's fight with reality plays similar havoc. In the presence of emotion, the mind fears loss of control. It reacts by suppressing emotional expression. But each emotion arises to pro-duce effective responses to life situations. The emotion is meant to play itself out, changing the situation; in response, another emotion arises. In other words, emotions naturally move and flow like a stream. When the mind suppresses the flow, it is as if a dam were built. Upstream, a lake of unexpressed emotion builds up, becoming bigger and more permanent than it would have been had it been allowed to simply flow unobstructed. Because emotions want to flow, the only way to keep an emotion around is to try not to have it.

In plant spirit medicine, we often find these emotional dams, or blocks, in people we're working with. Often the buildup of emotional energy produces physical symptoms, and it always produces crippling emotional problems. I say "crippling" because only through the emotions do we relate to the world. Imbalanced emotions create imbalanced relationships and actions. A person with a block of this kind cannot get really well, because a blockage at any point stops the flow everywhere.

To illustrate how this can play out, I give the example of an imaginary woman named Anne, who has pains in her gallbladder area. She says she's irritable and short-tempered with her husband and children. Five years ago, her father and two of her brothers died. Two years after that, her beloved cat passed away. She has not wept over any of her losses, but she is still putting food in her dead cat's dish every morning. Fear of grief has caused a block, and the unexpressed emotional energy is backed up, causing anger and abdominal pain. A plant spirit is called on to release the blockage, and Anne begins to sob deeply. At the next visit, she reports that she is getting along much better with her family and her pains are almost gone.

Since the mind is an expression of fear, you might suppose it gets along just fine with that emotion. Actually, though, the mind is even afraid of fear, and this is why it produces the "flight" part of the fight-or-flight response. The mind wants to be in control, lest some terrible loss should happen. It would be a terrible loss for the mind to see itself for what it is: simply an expression of fear that has important but limited usefulness. Even though the loss of self-importance is the much sought-after goal of spiritual practitioners everywhere, the mind runs and hides from fear. It hides from itself.

Where does the mind go? Where does it hide? It goes to a dissociated never-never land called "thinking." The mind claims that thinking is not emotional, but the claim is false. To be "in your head" means to be out of touch with your feelings, and to be out of touch with your feelings is to be out of touch with everybody and everything. Thinking is not emotionless; thinking is the mind running away in fear of confronting its own fear.

The mind can also run away into emotional numbness—a sense of not feeling anything. This dissociative trick is very similar to thinking. Like thinking, numbness is not neutral; it is not the absence of feeling. It is the unacknowledged presence of fear.

The direct experience of emotion cannot be explained or understood. It has no history, no future, no meaning. It is unpredictable, and it cannot be controlled. Therefore, the mind fears it.

Now we can answer the questions we posed earlier: If emotion is always present, why do we spend time and money watching movies that stir our feelings? Because even though emotion is present, it is heavily suppressed by the mind. Something in us needs to feel alive, and a good movie can fill the need, at least for a while. The aggression and violence in movies, the exploitation of sex and fear in them, show how much feeling has been dammed up, distorted, and overly amplified.

The next question was whether some of our actions are motivated by reason and logic rather than emotion. The answer is that reason and logic are not divorced from feeling; they are disguised forms of fear.

We can answer the third question—how can emotion be present when we feel blank?—the same way: emotion is present in blankness because blankness is just fear hiding in a somewhat different disguise.

If our tour of the landscape of fear seems bleak, you might be ready for some good news: there is bright, warm fire in the human heart. Connection, relationship, love, guidance, knowing, and transformation are some of the aspects of heart fire, but here we focus on the fire emotions: happiness and joy.

Happiness arises when a need or desire is fulfilled, as in this simple example: You are walking down the street feeling hungry for Chinese food. You see an attractive Chinese restaurant, and you go in. You order what you like. The food arrives; you find it delicious and satisfying. Your need/desire has been fulfilled, and you feel happy—until you get hungry again. Happiness depends on external circumstances, and since circumstances change quickly, happiness is meant to come and go quickly, like all emotions.

What I am calling "joy" is different, because it is independent of circumstances. Just as the nature of the sun is to shine, the nature of heart fire is joy. Nothing adds to it; nothing subtracts from it. It is a peaceful meta-emotion embracing everything. Like the sea, it is unaltered by waves of emotion arising and disappearing on its surface.

If this description makes joy seem illusory or out of reach, consider your experience going to the movies, where you find delight in laughter and tears, fear and anger, sympathy and grief. The only thing that keeps us from enjoying life as much as we enjoy the movies is the resistance to feeling our emotions in real time as much as we do in reel time. The medicine of the plant spirits softens the resistance.

Most of us consider happiness to be a desirable emotion. Sometimes we even think that the goal of life is to feel happy all the time. But happiness alone will not give us what we need to establish and maintain our boundaries. Growth is part of life, and to grow means to expand our boundaries. A seedling has small boundaries; the boundaries of a mature tree are much larger. It is the same in human life: a grownup has more extended boundaries than an infant. Our most obvious physical boundary is the surface of our skin. Should that boundary be violated, an emotion arises to restore it.

Let's say you are standing in line at the supermarket, and someone steps on your toe. If you realize the boundary violation was unintentional, the emotion you feel might not be very intense, and in response you might simply say, "Excuse me, but you stepped on my toe." This relatively modest emotional expression is sufficient to reestablish your physical boundary.

A stronger violation calls up a stronger boundary-setting expression. If you see that the person stepped on your foot on purpose, with the intention of bothering or hurting you, the emotion that arises will be more intense, as will your response. You might say, "Hey, get off me!" and push the person away. Whether the expression is mild, moderate, or strong, the emotion that maintains and restores boundaries is the same. It is called anger.

There are also boundaries beyond the purely physical ones. For example, let's say you manufacture widgets and you have a contract to deliver ten thousand of them to your customer by April 12. In order to do so, you have contracted with a supplier to deliver ten thousand widget switches by March 15, giving you enough time to install the switches in the widgets. But by April 12, the switches still have not arrived. You are unable to deliver the finished widgets your customer ordered, and they cancel the order. You have lost the $200,000 profit you stood to make on the deal, not to mention the trust of your customer and potential future customers. Your supplier has violated an agreed-upon boundary, and you feel angry. That emotion—anger—moves you to address the violation: you sue for breach of contract in order to compensate for your losses.

In itself, anger is a necessary and good thing because it motivates us to set proper boundaries. Anger becomes a problem only when it gets dammed up by fear.

People who know me realize I don't drink coffee, so they don't offer it (unless they are deliberately trying to annoy me). If someone unwittingly asks if I would like a cup, I simply say "No, thank you." This is a very mild expression of boundary setting. Technically it could be called anger, even though it is not aggressive. If I were afraid to decline the coffee, if I smiled and drank it every time it was offered, the pent-up energy would build and get out of proportion. Eventually I might respond to an innocent offer with real hostility or, just as bad, I might become angry and resentful toward myself. If this continued long enough it would rob me of my peace of mind and could even produce physical symptoms of illness.

Our society labels anger a negative emotion, which is to say we like to see it in the movies, but in real life we fear it. There is really no such thing as negative emotion; there is only natural emotion that can get over amplified and distorted through suppression, so that instead of leading us to set healthy, beneficial boundaries, anger can be distorted into aggression, hatred, and sickness.

Anger is not the only emotion that gets labeled as negative, as something to be shunned. A friend told me the psychotherapeutic profession recently classified grief as a pathology. This is truly tragic. Far from being an illness to be overcome, grief is a great, slow-moving healer to be welcomed with respect.

When you lose someone, Doctor Grief arrives at your home. He closes the doors and windows. He sits beside your bed and asks a hard question: "What is really important to you?"

He hears the answer in your weeping.

Another hard question: "Where is your strength?"

He sees your strength in your tears. He asks for more tears. And again, "More tears."

He washes you, again and again, in your tears.

"Will this never end?" you wonder.

Patiently, patiently, Doctor Grief cleanses your sorrow.

After what seems like eternities, he stands, bows with grave respect, and slowly walks out the door, which he leaves slightly ajar. On your doorstep, you see flowers and a brightly wrapped package with your name on it.

A mother puts a crying baby to her breast; a friend listens with understanding to someone talking about his problems; a caring person helps a homeless family; a neighbor brings a hot meal to a newly bereaved widow; someone considers how plants, animals, rocks, and waters feel about a development project; a group of leaders makes a decision by considering its effect on people seven generations later. Here we see sympathy at work, opening the door to a landscape of nurturance.

Sympathy does not get the bad press that is heaped on grief, fear, and anger; it is usually thought of as a noble emotion, which it is. But like the other emotions, it needs to move and flow. When fear blocks free expression, even sympathy gets unbalanced and problematic.

Fear says, "Smart people like me know there's not enough to go around, so you have to take care of Number One. If the idiots are having a hard time, it's their problem, not mine." Fear does not understand that sympathy feeds the giver as much as the receiver. Withholding sympathy only makes you hungrier, more competitive, more bent on taking care of yourself at any cost. This is how most people feel in today's workplaces. Men are particularly prone to this condition, although women are not exempt.

Women are a bit more likely to nurture everyone *except* Number One. Fear produces this distortion as well—a fear that somehow the self doesn't deserve to be cared for. As a result, others usually feel smothered and guilty while once again Number One goes hungry.

Our lives are lived in a stream of emotion, where free flow makes for good relationships and effective action—and for health itself. We humans are not the only ones in the stream; the plant beings live here too. They flow joyfully, and they can help us do the same.

chapter 8

PLACE

Many years ago, in the broad valley of the East Branch of the Delaware River, near what is now called Margaretville, New York, several Mohawk and Oneida families made camp for summer hunting and gathering.

One day an unrelated band came through the camp, and shortly afterward a dispute over territory arose between the two groups. A young warrior was soon found slain. Who was responsible for the killing? One group blamed the other, the other blamed the first, and they both suspected the third group. Accusations and counteraccusations were hurled. Tension and confusion built. Anger rose. War was at the point of breaking out, but they paused to consider: if they spent the short summer in battle, they would be unable to hunt and gather what they needed for the long winter.

The neighboring people to the west—the Onondagas—were known as the keepers of the council fires. The people determined to find an Onondaga medicine man and entreat him to come help them make peace.

The Onondagas were hard to locate, for they too were out hunting and gathering, but at length they found a medicine man named Tesakwanachee on his way back from pilgrimage in the Adirondacks to the north.

Tesakwanachee was young but of good reputation, so they explained their predicament and asked him to come to their camp, which he agreed to do.

He arrived to find the Mohawks claiming the camp as their territory and wanting the council fire to be held Mohawk style. The Oneidas were insisting on their own rules and authority. The two groups could not even agree how to sit around the fire and talk to each other.

The medicine man left the camp to take council with nearby forests, mountains, and waters. He was instructed to walk westward and then turn north into the first valley he would come to. There he was to walk along the stream, Saskawhihiwine, and watch for a sign in the water to show he had reached a sacred place where the spirit of the land would bring people together and resolve their differences.

He did as he was instructed. About a mile from the place where Saskawhihiwine joins the Delaware, Tesakwanachee saw a perfect circle in the pooled waters. This was the sign.

He returned to the camp and convinced the people to follow him to where the circle had appeared. He claimed it as neutral territory under Onondaga protocols. A council fire was built, the rift was healed, and peace was restored.

A council house was built on the site of the circle and used for many years as a special place to resolve conflict and produce healing. Even after it fell into disrepair, passersby would stop and honor the place with special offerings.

When Europeans pushed the indigenous peoples out, the place fell into a long slumber. Hundreds of years later, it reawakened, becoming the Blue Deer Center and headquarters of plant spirit medicine. Within a few months, the circle reappeared in the thin winter ice of Saskawhihiwine.

In this sacred story, the medicine man consulted the land in order to discover where to find peace and healing. He knew that *place* is more than an incidental backdrop; place has spirit, personality, and sacred purpose. Place is the starring actor in every drama, and without the star, the show can't go on.

The ancestors knew that some places produce strife and others produce peace. Some are good for hunting, others for growing crops. There are places to give birth and places to bury the dead. Settlements will flourish in some places, while others become sanctuaries for prayer and retreat.

The modern view is very different. We treat places as real estate, mere commodities for sale, to be used by the owners for any purpose they wish. But when owners' desires do not agree with the spirit of the place, the results can be failed enterprise, illness, and even death.

When it comes to plant spirit medicine, there is a similar divide between the ancestral view and the modern one. Today, plants are also seen as commodities. They are often forced to grow in places where they don't belong. Even though there may be helpful phytochemicals in the resulting herbal tinctures and capsules, the resentment of the plants can be there too.

Ancestral wisdom says *where* medicine grows is part of the medicine. Plants have roots; they belong to the land where they naturally come forth. They eat minerals and the remains of plants, animals, and humans. They eat the spirit and purpose of where they live. They embody and share the medicine of *place*.

chapter 9

SACRED PLANT TEACHERS

Colin Campbell, a *sangoma* and traditional African doctor from Botswana, tells the story of a villager in his country who fell seriously ill and called in a local traditional doctor for help. The healer examined the patient and then set off to consult with the mountains, waters, animals, and plants of the area. In a few days, he returned to announce his diagnosis: someone had cut down a tree without asking permission of the spirit of the tree itself. The disrespectful act of one person had created imbalance, which had showed up as someone else's illness. The villagers understood very well that there would be consequences for everyone unless good relationship to the trees could be restored. A ritual was prescribed to remediate the offense; the whole village participated, and the patient and his community returned to health.

This is not a story about an evil spirit out to smite people. Plant spirits are part of a web woven of love and respect, giving and receiving. We humans are part of it too. When we tear the web, a messenger comes to town carrying a suitcase full of something designed to make sure we take the message to heart. The suitcase is labeled "misfortune."

"For the sake of all creation, repair the web," the messenger says. "Get back to what supports you, what supports others, what supports everything: love and respect, giving and receiving."

This story should be remembered in any interaction with plants. If you are interested in engaging one of the sacred plant teachers, such as peyote, ayahuasca, or special mushrooms, you should remember the story as if your life depends on it. The power of these plants is beyond imagination; you don't want to see *their* messenger arriving with his suitcase.

Some will say, "I have good intentions, and I am respectful. There won't be any problems for *me.*" This is naïve. Yes, sometimes naïve engagements work out okay, but sometimes they don't. If we wish to be blessed with knowledge, wisdom, or healing, what must we give in return? How must we demonstrate our respect? It is not for us to say. The spirit of the plant will make the call.

To understand respectful engagement with these great teachers, we have to go back to the time when the gods were singing a great story—the story of the world. Their singing brought the world and all its creatures into being, including, eventually, us humans.

The Darwinians made their best guess about how this came about, but according to the indigenous wisdom keepers, they didn't get it quite right. The different human peoples did not evolve out of a common ancestor; they were each born out of the womb of their own homeland. We appeared in different parts of the world at the same time. Each group was as much a part of their environment as the other animals and plants of the region.

The Arctic willow and the banana have much in common: they both have roots and leaves, they both do photosynthesis, and so on. At the same time, each is part of a different environment and needs different conditions to live and thrive. The Inuit and the indigenous Amazonian are as similar and as different as the Arctic willow and the banana.

Each of the animals was sung into the world with the equipment it needs: wings, gills, fur, pointy or hooked beak, claws, fast-running legs, a keen sense of smell or hearing, and so on. The special equipment given to us was the human mind with its unique ability to create the sensation of separateness: "This is me, and everything else is not me." The mind goes on from this primal separation to make many more separations and distinctions: "This is a rock. That is a plant. That is a stick."

Our mind, driven by a fearful concern for survival, comes up with creative interventions: "I am hungry, and the deer runs faster than I do. If I break the rock to make a sharp point and fasten it to the stick with plant fibers, I can throw it at the deer and have a meal."

All this is fine, but a problem arises when we dwell too much in the mind. The mind creates the illusion of a separate self and then justifies any action it thinks will protect that self. Like the man who cut down the tree for his own selfish purposes, we tear the web of relatedness. This brings many misfortunes: illness, isolation, never-ending fear, personal and environmental catastrophe.

Human intelligence is amnesiac. It forgets that we are part of the web of being, and this forgetfulness is the source of illness and suffering. For this reason, when we were given this problematic gift, we were also given the ways to keep it in balance as a small, though important, part of our lives. All the original peoples were given teachings and practices to remind us that we are part of the web. Remembering produces healing, wisdom, a flourishing environment, and a sustainable way of life.

Some peoples were given sacred plant teachers as memory aids—doorways to sacred realms of knowledge, wisdom, and healing. Some of these plants, like peyote, are ingested; others, like the Wind Tree, are not. But not one of them was brought forth everywhere. This is because, as we have seen, peoples are different. The Inuit and the Amazonian, the Aborigine and the Celt, the Zulu and the Mongol each have different needs. Their souls are made of the ancestral stuff of different lands. The ways of remembering are different for each. None of the sacred plant teachers are for everybody.

In the old days, it was perfectly clear who could benefit from a sacred plant teacher. For example, if you were a member of a group that had been through countless cycles of living and dying where the ayahuasca vine grows, then you and ayahuasca were made for each other. If you were from someplace else, ayahuasca was not for you.

These days it is more difficult to know whether something is for you. The collapse of adequate funerary rites has caused many souls to wander after death and drift into foreign ancestral realms, so the reservoirs of ancestral energy have become quite mixed. Since the human soul is constructed from ancestral energy, we ourselves have become soul mutts. To say it another way, your genealogy and place of birth are no longer reliable guides to what your soul is made of. Maybe you were born in Chicago into Eastern-European Jewish families, as I was. Despite that, maybe your soul is mostly made of Huichol ancestral stuff, as mine is. If so, maybe you could benefit from peyote, as I have. But do you really know the construct of your own soul? In these times, few people do.

When you consider working with a sacred plant teacher, do you consider whether the plant sees you as one of its people—the people it was brought into the world to help? Or do you consider only what *you* want? If it's all about *you,* then the plant teacher will see you as disrespectful. It may ignore you, it may play a little trick on you, or it may send its messenger with a bulging suitcase.

These days, you always need the help of a trustworthy guide who can look into your soul to see whether you and the sacred plant teacher are soul mates and to help you walk the plant's path; actually, the sacred plants insist on it. They were brought into the world to benefit us. They open into vastness we cannot navigate on our own. On our own, we easily get lost, and lost people are of no benefit to themselves or others, except as an example of what not to do.

A good guide has herself had a guide. She has walked the path and is still walking it. She knows the direction, the twists and turns. She knows who belongs to the medicine and who does not. She has seen many who have received blessings and some who have suffered misfortune. The successful ones, like her, stayed true to the traditions given by the plant and passed down through generation after generation of ancestors. The unsuccessful ones wanted to have it *their* way.

In the Huichol tradition, this is what it takes to become a guide for peyote: First, there is at least five years of grueling apprenticeship under the supervision of a tricky, hardball-playing shaman. Then there is a dangerous initiation ritual. If the candidate makes it through initiation successfully, he has himself become a shaman and must take on a life of service to his community. But even then he is not ready to guide others. He must work as a shaman for another five years. If he is seen to be an effective healer who is devoted to his people's welfare, he may ask for a second initiation, which is even more dangerous than the first. After running that gauntlet, he presents himself for a third initiation as a guide to peyote. In that final initiation, the ancestors, the gods, and peyote itself at last declare the shaman ready to help others who would ask this sacred plant teacher for help.

The training and initiation are different for different sacred plants and different peoples, but preparing to become a guide is always a big responsibility. The one who disregards tradition, who looks for shortcuts, who merely declares him- or herself a guide—that person is a dangerous fool.

These days all kinds of people offer themselves. Some are authentic; some are deluded; some are after money, sex, or power. Make sure your guide is properly initiated and has your interest at heart.

When the moment arrives to invoke the medicine of the sacred plant teacher, ask yourself, what kind of situation is the sacred plant teacher invited into? Is it focused, respectful and safe, as the plant desires? Or is it scattered, contaminated by egotism—an invitation to misfortune? A trustworthy human guide follows the instructions given to the ancestors about how to build a proper ritual container, and he listens carefully for guidance on moment-to-moment adjustments.

The rituals of engagement are not invented by an individual; they are not even invented by a culture. They were given to the peoples along with the plant; actually, they are part of the sacred presence of the plant.

When the people of the peyote, the Huichols, want to ask their sacred plant teacher for special gifts, they take great care with the ritual setting. First the human guide sets a date for a pilgrimage to the birthplace of their traditions. There is a preparatory month of abstinence from sex, salt, and bathing. A deer is hunted and killed with the proper prayers and respect; a bull is also purchased and properly sacrificed. Special offerings are constructed and prayed over with love and devotion; later these will be left at the sacred site. The journey from the Huichol village to the birthplace is long—until a few years ago, it took a month of walking. These days, trucks and buses can be hired, but the cost is so great that the journey may be postponed for lack of funds. Along the way, there is much protocol to attend to, culminating at the entrance to the holy land with a specific purification rite that leaves the fasting pilgrims innocent as young children. There are moments to move and moments to stay still, moments to speak and moments to keep silent. A fire is built, consecrated, and lovingly tended. An altar is constructed, festooned with offerings, and anointed with the blood of the deer and the bull. The sacred medicine is prayed to, searched for, found, prayed to again and again, blessed by the attending shaman, and finally eaten. The prayers, the offerings, the altar preparation—everything is done with scrupulous and loving attention to the instructions given to the Ancestors at the beginnings of time. The pilgrims vigil through the night. At dawn they sing the traditional prayers of gratitude and start the long journey back to their village.

Traditional indigenous peoples understand such practices; they know the practical value of rituals, and they take great care with them. Modern Western people often feel these things are quaint and obsolete. But have we benefited from our "highly evolved" approach? I know many traditional people—grounded, practical, and effective community leaders, farmers, healers, artists—who make wonderful contributions to life as a way of sharing the gifts they receive from their sacred plants. How many Westerners do you know who produce blessings for others from their involvement with sacred plant teachers?

Due to their enormous popularity, two sacred plant teachers deserve special mention here: marijuana and tobacco. Let's consider marijuana first. Its homeland is Central Asia. In the Western world, it is rare to find a person with substantial soul relatedness to that land and plant. It is even more rare to find someone initiated into its indigenous protocols, and it's rarer still to find a properly initiated guide willing to teach others. Marijuana tricks people into believing they are benefiting from it. Outside of its sacred context, the sacred plant teacher becomes a trickster carrying an intriguing, prettily decorated suitcase.

Many more people have relatedness to tobacco, but very few recognize and respect its sacredness. These days it is feared and condemned as a poison, and the numbers of smoking-related deaths and illnesses would seem to support that view. But tobacco, like all sacred plants, becomes destructive only when treated with disrespect. The statistics do not prove the malevolence of this plant; they only demonstrate that it is massively abused.

Yet the plant that produces danger and illness in the modern world produces healing and protection in the indigenous world. Tobacco was brought forth in the Americas, and I have never been anywhere on these continents where it does not have an important place in indigenous spiritual practices. It helps people hear with the ears of the heart, so it is a special adjunct to prayer and the source of many blessings. In most cultures, tobacco does not require elaborate conditions for its proper use, but it does demand unfailing gratitude and respect. A minimal ritual setting is good for keeping the user focused and honest about his or her intentions.

Lest you think these sacred plant teachers have no relevance in today's "real" world, consider this: A few years ago, I was talking to a Huichol acquaintance. He was a prosperous man by Huichol standards, and he was serving a term of unpaid community service as the traditional governor of his area. He spoke excellent, educated Mexican Spanish. To make conversation, I asked him if he had attended a nearby Catholic mission school, where others of his generation had learned Spanish.

"No," he said. "I never went to school. I don't know how to read or write."

Surprised, I asked him, "So how did you learn to speak Spanish so well?"

"I learned the same way my grandfather did. He was a great shaman who lived to be 110 years old. He learned Spanish at about 80."

"Well, how did your grandfather learn?"

"Peyote taught him."

chapter 10

An Ordinary Life

I was born in Chicago and grew up in Winnipeg and San Francisco. My father worked as a manager for various businesses, and my stepmother was a housewife. My upbringing was conventional in every respect, down to the divorce of my parents when I was eight years old. As a youngster, I was sickly and intellectual and had no feeling of kinship with nature. In fact, my allergies to pollen led me to dread plants as the enemy.

While I was a graduate student in filmmaking during the late 1960s, one day I realized I knew nothing about the earth I lived on. It suddenly seemed urgent that I find out, so I left the university for a farm in Vermont. On the farm, my ignorance led me into one problem after another, but I enjoyed farm life nevertheless. I found a satisfying lesson in each new difficulty. Especially satisfying were my experiences with herbal medicine.

I started practicing herbalism because of a cranky old goat named Eloise. When Eloise got an eye infection one day, I took her to a veterinarian, who pronounced there was no cure for her. He assured me she was going to die, but offered a prescription anyway. I thanked him, took the prescription, and left. When I got home, I tossed the prescription into the trash and decided that since the vet couldn't help, I might as well try to treat Eloise myself. I looked up her ailment in a book of veterinary herbalism. The recommended herbs were growing on my farm, so I picked them and dosed her according to the instructions. Within a few days, she was her normal self again. Her disease had completely disappeared.

After a few more successes, I discovered I had a passion for natural healing, and I wanted to make a profession of it. In order to do so, I needed a teacher, but I had no idea how to go about finding a teacher or even whether such a person actually existed. One day, my neighbors in Vermont told me about their friend Diane, who had contracted a mysterious disease in Asia and traveled extensively trying to find someone who could heal her. Everywhere she went, she heard stories of a great acupuncturist named J. R. Worsley. Since none of the practitioners she consulted had been able to help, she went to consult Worsley at his home in England. The Englishman quickly removed Diane's illness and brought her to a wonderful state of health she had never experienced before. Diane was so impressed that she stayed on to study with Worsley.

This story gave me faith that the kind of teacher I needed did exist after all and that I would surely find him. I left the farm to start looking. Three years and many disappointments later, I finally did find my first teacher. He turned out to be none other than J. R. Worsley himself!

I first heard Worsley speak at a seminar. He was teaching about the Chinese medical tradition of the Five Elements, and he was simultaneously funny, down to earth, and profound. His medicine affirmed everything I had learned on the farm and promised to teach everything I wanted to know. I forgot about my local weeds and went to England to learn what I could about acupuncture.

Chinese medicine, as I discovered, attributes healing to the balance of natural energies. In classical times, Chinese physicians placed great emphasis on the mind and spirit, and these realms were within the province of Worsley acupuncture. In keeping with tradition, Worsley held that the earth and its creatures are made of the same energy that turns the wheel of the seasons. In fact, he said, the seasons mold human nature. Each of the Five Elements corresponds to a season, and the energies of these seasons nurture and sustain us in different ways.

Hot summertime energy shows up in the structures that maintain our temperature: sweat glands, heart, circulatory system, and the metabolic fire in each cell. Physical survival depends on the right amount of heat, and heat is also essential to our minds. When we warm up to others, we know joy. Our spirit thrives on the warmth and joy that give meaning to life.

Indian summer is the fifth or extra season. At this time of year, Mother Nature offers a sweet, bountiful harvest that provides the body with food, the mind with understanding, and the spirit with a sympathy that can respond to the needs of others. Nourishment is prepared and delivered by the stomach, spleen and pancreas, and breasts.

As the old year wanes, in autumn, the crisp air announces the beginning of something new. The lungs take in fresh inspiration and guidance while the colon gets rid of grudges, hurts, sorrows, feelings of unworthiness, and feces. Autumn teaches us to value what we have and to grieve for what we have lost.

Winter is a time of inner quiet that puts us at the wellspring of will and ambition. While nature sleeps, the rain and snow fill the earth's reservoirs with water, the fluid of life. Our kidneys and bladder control the fluids that keep body, mind, and spirit flowing. Winter enables us to know fear and awe.

Spring is a burst into the future, a time for creatures to be born and grow. This time is not over when our bodies reach full stature. We must keep growing all our lives, or else we become stunted, frustrated, and angry. The organizers of our growth are the liver and gallbladder.

The five seasonal energies, or Five Elements, are the stuff of which everyone and everything is made. Classical Chinese medicine teaches that the balance of these energies is health and that imbalance is illness. The goal of healing is to restore natural harmony. When this is done, symptoms will disappear automatically, since they are only messengers of imbalance.

Chinese medicine notes that the state of a person's elements can be detected by observing the emotions. There are several ways to detect a person's emotions. An animal can tell precisely how a person feels by noting their scent, and as a student of acupuncture, I learned to recover the use of my nose so that I too could smell people's feelings. Emotions also have color. I learned to perceive the subtle but distinct hue that each emotion lends to the complexion.

Emotions also make sound. When we are feeling sympathetic, for example, our voices become quite musical, whereas when we are angry, we make harsher sounds. Infants who do not yet understand words are able to interpret the sound of the voice perfectly well, but as an adult I had to resensitize myself to these nuances.

And emotions throb with the heartbeat. Following classical Chinese medical procedure, I learned to feel the arterial pulse in twelve different locations in order to get detailed information about the balance of the elements.

Professor Worsley also educated me in the ways of the spirit. On one occasion, he spent a classroom week talking about the spirit, and on the last day, he offered an experience of what he had been talking about. One by one, he invited each student to come to the front of the class and receive acupuncture treatment for the spirit. Before long, one man was laughing uncontrollably, while another was slumped in a corner with a dazed look on his face. A young woman was chuckling happily as tears streamed down her face, and another was sobbing and screaming. Worsley's needles had touched the spirit of each student, and each had been transformed by the experience.

When the professor needled me, I felt rivulets of sparkling energy flowing through my body. After the feeling wore off, I did not notice any further change. I reflected on the acupuncture points he had used on me, and I recalled that those points were useful for mending energies shattered by trauma. This puzzled me, because I was in love and there were no traumas in sight at that time. The next day I flew home, and my loved one greeted me with the news that our affair was over. This caused me great pain, but I was not shattered by the blow because I had already been treated for it.

In England I began to appreciate how nature fulfills human life. I saw that when nature is out of balance, we feel a longing that drives everything about us, including our thoughts, feelings, tastes, cravings, voice, skin color, and odor. Most importantly, longing distorts our experience of life. Our symptoms merely dramatize the true disease, the need of our soul.

I began my practice full of enthusiasm and ready to bring summer sun, harvest sweetness, autumn inspiration, winter peace, and spring rebirth into the hearts of my patients through acupuncture. During the early years, I thought a lot about Professor Worsley's teaching on herbalism, which he used to deliver in one sentence: "Anything that can be done with needles can also be done with herbs. But if you use herbs, for God's sake use local ones because they are not ten times stronger, they are not a hundred times stronger, they are *one thousand times stronger* than plants that grow someplace else." I liked this teaching. I did not know why local plants were stronger, and I had no idea how plants could heal the spirit.

Professor Worsley didn't seem to have a clue either. I believe he was speaking purely from intuition, and my intuition told me he was right.

In July of 1980, after a year teaching at Worsley's College of Traditional Acupuncture in England, I was on an airplane returning to California. Somewhere over Canada's Northwest Territories I made a promise to myself: "I am going to revive the use of local plants to heal the spirit." It was a rash pledge. I had nothing to support it with except youthful idealism, but since I was youthful and idealistic, I took it seriously.

Arriving in Santa Barbara, I began to search for sources of information about medicinal uses of local wild plants. Herbal literature was no help because it was based on European and East Coast American plants. Inquiries with local Native American people were also fruitless because Chumash herbal lore had nearly disappeared as a result of cultural genocide.

With no outside authorities to turn to, I resolved to use my own mind. Chinese medicine provided me with a set of correspondences, which I decided to apply to plants in order to figure out their properties. For example, Indian summer energy gives rise to the yellow color, the sweet taste, and the stomach's capacity for digestion. The first plant I considered was common fennel, *Foeniculum vulgare*. This plant puts out yellow flowers in Indian summer. Every part of the plant is intensely sweet, and it has a reputation as a tonic to the stomach and digestion. This plant was obviously saturated with Indian summer energy. If this was the first success of my analytical method, though, it was also the last. Every other plant I studied had a mishmash of conflicting correspondences; the color corresponded to one season, the taste to a second, and the time of its appearance to a third. It became clear I was not going to get what I wanted this way, and I didn't know how to fulfill my pledge. I needed a new approach, and since I had no idea of what that might be, I decided to shelve the whole project.

By this time I had made my first visit to don José Ríos (Matsuwa), the Huichol Indian shaman in Mexico. The experience, as I recounted in chapter 3, made a deep impression on me. I sensed that learning more about shamanism might help me with my work, but I did not know any practical way of getting shamanic training.

Within a few months, I was approached by an acquaintance who wanted acupuncture treatment for some health problems. Instead of paying with money, she proposed to pay by teaching me something she thought I would find interesting. I barely knew this woman and had no idea what she wanted to teach, but I instinctively accepted her offer. I soon confirmed that my instinct was accurate. As a young girl, she had discovered she could leave her body and journey beyond limitations of time and space, acquiring knowledge and capacities as she went. In any case, this learning to journey among the dream worlds was the something she thought I would find interesting. I worked with her for about a year, deepening my knowledge of acupuncture and exploring other areas of interest to both of us. It never occurred to me to apply this method to learning about plants.

After we parted company, I still had a yen to learn something about shamanism. I heard that the American anthropologist Michael Harner was teaching some shamanistic techniques in a weekend course, so I traveled to New York to study with him. I was delighted to find out that my previous year had already given me a bit of experience. I was also happy with Michael's course. It was clear he had more to teach, so I signed up for further study.

It was Michael who suggested a technique for contacting plant spirits that was precisely the new approach I needed to fulfill my pledge. English plantain, the first plant I contacted, assured me the plant spirits would be happy to teach me and had, in fact, been waiting for almost two hundred years in the hope someone would ask for their help in healing the human spirit.

After that first contact, I took advantage of every spare hour to learn from the plants of my region. I had already learned their language—the language of the five seasons. The plant spirits gave me knowledge I could immediately put into practice, and put it into practice I did, gingerly at first, but with more confidence as I saw evidence that it worked. Within a few months, I had amassed a body of plant lore that would have taken generations to acquire any other way.

While I have been blessed with exceptional teachers, my story is unexceptional in every other way. I had a middle-class childhood with the usual amount of suffering and insecurities. I was trained by my parents in the rational materialism of the day, and I was not initiated into any indigenous tradition until many years after I rediscovered the medicine of the plant spirits. Over the years, I have come to honor my ordinariness and to consider it a testament to what can be accomplished by a person with no resources other than a dogged interest in healing.

part two

My Plant
Spirit Dream

chapter 11

FIRE

The sun, thin and weak with age, has finished its short journey across the sky. Underfoot, ice crystals grow amid blackened stems. The few remaining birds have tucked their heads under their wings; there is nothing to sing about. Among all the creatures, only the People are happy and talkative. The icy blackness does not penetrate the circle of the campfire where they sit, sharing the adventures of the day. They rejoice in good fortune and laugh off the bad, for they have the pleasure of shared warmth.

Young mothers are tucking in their babies. The bigger children sit at Storyteller's knees, eagerly awaiting one of his tales.

Storyteller looks at the expectant little faces. He chuckles. He places two logs on the fire. "Thank you, older brother," he says.

One of the children raises her voice. "Storyteller, why do you always talk to the firewood and call it 'older brother'?"

The adults laugh. They know this question is sure to be answered with the story of "Why the Sun Has to Rest at Night." This is a complicated tale involving some of Storyteller's best characters: Bear, Trout, and Blackberry Bush.

The story begins and continues into the night, punctuated by giggles and guffaws. One by one, the children drop off to sleep, and when the telling is over, Storyteller allows himself a few last chuckles as he banks the fire. His wife approaches, wiping tears of laughter from her cheeks. She smiles an invitation to him. In her eyes, he sees the glowing red coals.

In this scenario, the campfire gathered the people, warmed them, and brought out their mirth. It is a scene as old as humanity, repeated countless times all over the world, for humans have always lived by the fire, cooking and eating, talking and laughing, caring for children, and listening to wise elders. Today, fire is encased in metal and plastic and is controlled with dials and thermostats, yet it is still in our kitchens, our furnaces, our vehicles, and our electric devices. But where are the people? Are they looking into each other's eyes, or are they looking at screens? Do they know each other's joys and cares? Do they feel they belong to each other and the place they live?

When I was a boy living in a white, middle-class neighborhood, people lived pretty isolated lives, yet kids played together in the streets. We roamed freely in and out of each other's houses, often eating together or sleeping over. Parents socialized with each other from time to time. On the other hand, fifty years later, I lived in a place that had become typical in the United States. I couldn't call it a neighborhood, because after living there for fifteen years, I did not know anyone's name. Neither children nor adults were seen on the streets unless they were in cars.

One blessed day, we had a power outage. Within minutes people came out of their homes onto the street, bringing children, card tables, board games, guitars, gossip, singing, and laughter. After a couple of hours, power was restored, and people went back to their computers and televisions, leaving the area as desolate as before.

If we look at the world around us, we see fire everywhere. Plants capture heat and light from the sun and store it in their flesh. When we eat plants and the animals who eat plants, we absorb that stored-up heat and light, which powers every heartbeat, every step we take. Each of our cells is like a tribe gathered around its metabolic campfire. We live by the fire in our own bodies.

Science says heat is the movement of molecules: faster movement equals higher temperature; slower movement is lower temperature. An object with no movement at all would be at "absolute zero" temperature, but this is only a theoretical abstraction, because without movement an object would not be able to exchange with anything around it, and without exchange, nothing can exist.

If this seems like an extravagant claim, consider the example of a tree, which breathes out the oxygen vital to animals. Animals return the favor by breathing out the carbon dioxide vital to the tree. The droppings and decaying carcasses of animals feed the soil, which nourishes the growth of leaves, which in turn feed the animals. The tree, through its roots, takes up life-sustaining water. Through the leaves, the moisture returns to the sky so it can fall on the earth once again as rain. There are other exchanges as well, but if even one of these cycles is interrupted, the tree perishes. It becomes dead wood, whose cycles of exchange with soil, air, plants, and animals are carried out through a complex process called decay. When decay is complete, what was once a tree will have turned into moist, rich earth and a multitude of small and large life-forms. New trees sprout and grow; the exchange cycles go on. Everything owes its existence to cycles of exchange. Some forms last longer than others, but there are no discrete objects in the world. We are all simply focuses of exchange. When exchange is over, we get recycled.

There is a beautiful word for the exchange that makes us part of everything: the word is *love*. Exchange, relationship, joy, love—it's all fire making the world go around, conducting the orchestra of the world.

The ancient Chinese sages likened our fire to an enlightened emperor who controls all the activities in the empire of body, mind, and spirit. They called this fire "the Supreme Controller." *Supreme* referred to the Divine, which, they knew, does not control with force or fear; it controls with love. That love lives in us as our heart.

Some time ago, I was consulted by a fifty-year-old man whose heart had been cold for so many years he could no longer find the enthusiasm to do anything. He just collected unemployment and puttered around the house amid a clutter of unfinished projects. I gave this man a plant spirit to warm him and give him the heart to take the helm of his life once more. His face flushed pink. The next day he phoned to say he was burning up, and he hadn't stopped crying since the night before. Was there anything I could do to turn down the heat? I assured him both the heat and the sadness would soon pass and he would feel much better afterward.

The man phoned again the following day with new enthusiasm in his voice. He had some things to talk to me about and invited me to meet for dinner. His chat over dinner was full of purpose and vigor. The day before, he had taken the steps to close a major business deal that had been blocked for months. He had also phoned the nearby university with instructions on how to bring to fruition one of his inventions that had been languishing in the laboratory for years. The invention, significantly, consisted of an instrument and surgical technique to clear out blockages in the arteries of the heart.

Fire naturally produces joy, happiness, pleasure, laughter, relationship, and sexuality. The sages knew these gifts of fire provide protection from fear, heaviness, and taking things to heart. They spoke of this aspect of fire as the official in charge of the Pleasures of the People. It is also sometimes called the "heart protector."

When the heart protector is healthy, we can laugh at ourselves and our difficulties. We take pleasure in our warm relationships with others. We have satisfying sexual encounters. When the official is out of balance, we can feel cold, isolated, terribly vulnerable, untrusting, and bitter. Our lives may be consumed with the effort to deny or compensate for this suffering.

The heart protector does not correspond to an organ. You cannot point it out in a cadaver. For this reason, conventional medical doctors are unlikely to take it seriously. Nevertheless, it is as real as the nose on your face. Maybe it's more real, because you can't go to a plastic surgeon and get a heart-protector job!

Charlotte, one of my students, had a particularly vivid experience of what can happen when the heart protector gets the warmth it needs after years of deprivation. Here's what she wrote about the experience:

> I was skeptical before I started treatment. I had no idea what
> to expect, but when I received the first plant spirit, I instantly
> dropped into a deep state of consciousness, and I saw a spirit in
> front of me. I knew it was a plant spirit.[3] At the second [stage of
> the treatment] I heard Chopin playing. It was as if he were pres-
> ent in the room, as if I were inside the piano. It was so beautiful!
> When you gave me the third plant spirit, an angel appeared to

me. I felt great. I felt a lot of energy move up into my chest. That night I had important dreams.

I felt elated for about fourteen hours, and then the work of cleaning things out started. On a physical level, I had to poop constantly for days. That was okay, but the emotional work was pretty devastating. I started to go through my characteristic hurt behavior. You asked me to demonstrate something in front of class, and I couldn't do it. I was overwhelmed by old feelings: not being good enough, being betrayed, being ostracized from the group, not being part of the group, retreating inside to some place where I "knew better, anyway." This exacerbated not belonging. Since it's "better" not to belong, let's stay not belonging. Even though I was experiencing this, I was also watching it. I knew I had felt like this all my life. I was getting to my deepest symptoms of aloneness and sorrow.

I went through hell for twelve hours. I had all of the worst memories from my life: the alienation and betrayal in the music business, the hurt I went through when I left my spiritual community and seventy-five of my closest friends never even called to find out why I wasn't there any more. As a child, I went through that all the time. I was never able to belong. There were times that night when I even felt like killing myself. It's strange to say this, but I feel I was able to move through this quickly because the treatment was sustaining me somehow.

The next day in class, we made a dream journey to Fire. When I got to the heart protector, I saw a huge, open wound just ripped apart.[4]

I began to piece together that this wound was a spiritual wound: not belonging, not feeling that I could trust. It had been repeated over and over in my life. My cynicism, my criticalness—I could see that these were my defenses, my protection from the pain of not belonging.

On the third day, I had the courage to state to the class what I was feeling. This was a big leap of trust. It enabled me to belong. I wouldn't have been able to do that before.

Since then, I've noticed dramatic differences. I'm able to go into new situations. When we got back from the plant spirit medicine class, I went to the first meeting of a dance class I had signed up for. When I arrived, there were about a hundred people in the room. I panicked. "This is too many people! Let's get out of here!" But I was able to stay, participate, and even enjoy the class. I know that for some people this would be insignificant, but for me it was a really big deal to feel protected enough to participate like that.

I've been to L.A. and New York; I just feel totally at ease wherever I go. With each treatment, I feel a vital essence is being restored to me. Each time it strengthens a little more. It's a little easier to trust. Also, I've become sexually interested again for the first time in years—a big difference! Here's another thing: I never have to wear blush anymore. Everyone thinks my skin looks radiant. No one in New York can believe that I'm not wearing makeup. I'm glowing from the inside out.

I'm much less self-conscious about my body. Years of therapy about body image have not been as fruitful as a few plant spirit medicine treatments. It's not so much that my body is changing, although I have lost weight. It's more that I have buoyancy, a resilience inside, so that life doesn't feel despairing. I know that I'll never have to go through that despair again. Now I have more vitality and more ability to do what I want to do.

It's not as if you get treated by a plant spirit and immediately you drop thirty pounds, although I suppose that could happen. It's as if the care and nurturing that you're looking for in whatever your drug is—whether it's food or shopping or alcohol—you're getting that from the inside now.

At the time of the summer solstice, the sun's longest journey across the sky, there is a huge festival in Santa Barbara, California. At noon a parade starts down the main street, which is lined by everyone in town who isn't in the parade itself. The parade is dedicated to the sun, to summer, and most of all to fun. The goal of each float is to make people happy. Outlandish costumes, grotesque monsters, ten-foot-tall clowns, samba dancers on stilts, jugglers on roller skates, block-long serpents, pantomime artists, and jazzy bands heighten the festivity. When the parade is over, the participants and spectators walk to a nearby park, where they spend the rest of the day feasting and dancing.

Santa Barbara's Solstice Festival is entirely noncommercial. There is no advertising of any kind. No one gets paid for the huge tasks of organizing and preparing for the event. Why is it so unusual to have a large public celebration with no profit motive? The answer has to do with fire, sex, and spirit.

It doesn't take much subtlety to get the connection between fire and sex: "Come on, baby, light my fire." Fire is what gives us pleasure. Let's have a quick look at how we're doing with respect to sexual warmth. On the physical level, we're plagued with problems. Impotence, frigidity, and premature ejaculation cause marital strains. Among unmarried adults, teens, and preteens, pregnancy and sexually transmitted diseases are huge problems. If we are enjoying sexual pleasure at all, it seems it is only with the wrong people at the wrong times. On the mental level, sex is used to sell alcohol, cigarettes, coffee, milk, automobile tires, electronic equipment, vinyl siding, and more.

We are looking for the hot stuff because our spirits are cold. Did our parents and teachers make it their job to warm our spirits? Most likely, the people who did are the ones who now stand out in our memories. We have only one institution that even recognizes the human spirit and that is the church, but our churches are dour and solemn. Where are our temples of divine laughter?

What brings warmth and pleasure to our spirit? No amount of sleeping around can do it. Romance doesn't do it either. Bombing Baghdad didn't help. The only thing that can warm us is love. We live in a cold-hearted society. We are spiritually frigid, and so we have an infantile craving for pleasure. This craving is whipped into a frenzy by purveyors of merchandise of every kind. If we had a healthier relationship to fire and the sun, every town in the nation might have innocent noncommercial celebrations. But because our pleasures are so contaminated by the profit motive, the Santa Barbara Solstice Festival is quite unusual.

Observing the action of the sun on growing plants, the ancient Chinese maintained that fire has the power to bring things to maturity. A mature human being is one whose spirit has been warmed by the fire of love.

People from mature societies like the Hopi have some penetrating observations about our own culture. Fred Coyote tells the story of an anthropologist who went to a Hopi elder to record some of his people's songs:

The old man took him out on the edge of the mesa and he sang a song. The "anthro" was recording and making notes, and he said, "What is that song about?"

The old [Hopi] man said, "Well, that's about when the kachinas came down into the mountains and then the thunderheads built up around the San Francisco peaks, and then we sing and those clouds come out across the desert and it rains on the gardens and we have food for our children."

And the old man sang him another song. And the "anthro" said, "What was that song about?"

The old man answered, "That song was about when my wife goes down to the sacred spring to get water to prepare food for us and to prepare the medicines—because without that sacred spring we wouldn't live very long."

And so it went all afternoon. Every time the old man would sing a song, the "anthro" would say, "What's that about?" And the old man would explain it. It's about something or other—a river, rain, water.

Eventually this anthropologist was getting a little short-tempered. He said, "Is water all you people sing about down here?"

And the old man said, "Yes." He explained: "For thousands of years in this country we [Hopi] have learned to live here. Because our need for this water is so great to our families and to our people and to our nations, most of our songs are about our greatest need. I listen to a lot of American music. Seems like most American music is about love." He asked, "Is that why? Is that because you don't have very much?"[5]

Adelle was an attractive professional woman of middle years who came to me for plant spirit medicine. She smiled easily and laughed a lot and was successful, well liked, and happily married. Her laughter had a slight edge, but she was so vivacious that no one would have guessed she complained of fatigue.

Looking at Adelle's face, I noticed a subtle ashen color—a lack of normal healthy ruddiness. (A healthy red color has nothing to do with exposure to the sun. It comes from the flush of joy and pleasure within.) I discreetly sniffed the odor of her body, which smelled scorched—like burnt toast. Laughter predominated in the sound of her voice even as she spoke of unhappy things. She presented herself as a joyful person, but the joy was forced. I inferred that in the past she had been treated with coldness and indifference and had felt unloved and heartbroken. She had been working so hard to appear cheerful that she had tired herself out. Her fire was burning low.

I invoked the spirit of foothill penstemon for Adelle. Foothill penstemon has a beautiful fuchsia-and-blue flower that makes anyone happier just to look at. The spirit of this plant brings joy but is not a narcotic. It makes you work to clear out heartache. After receiving the penstemon spirit, Adelle closed her eyes and volunteered that she felt a pleasant sensation that appeared "blue and fuschia" in color. I checked her pulses. The response was very good, so I ended the treatment and asked her to return in a week.

Nothing unusual happened to Adelle until the next day. Around noon, she came down with a fever and flulike symptoms and went home to bed. She was lying with her eyes closed when she began to relive a long-forgotten scene from many years before. She was a teenage girl lying in bed, her body was covered with painful welts, and she had cramping in her abdomen such as she had never felt before. Suddenly her mother strode into the room, looked at her, and said, "You feel bad because you are about to become a woman, and that's what being a woman is—pain and suffering!" Without another word, her mother wheeled around and strode out of the room. Adelle the teenager—and Adelle the woman of the present—cried brokenheartedly. How could her mother have been so cold and indifferent?

Just as the sorrow was beginning to subside, Adelle found herself reliving another moment of heartbreak: the death of her father. This trauma was followed by another and another. In all, Adelle spent three hours in bed weeping. Afterward she felt shaken, but well enough to get up. The flu symptoms were gone.

In the days that followed, she felt extraordinarily well. Colors appeared vivid and intense. Food tasted like ambrosia. Music moved her to tears. Sex was ecstatic. Her relationship with her husband reached new heights. Her complaints about fatigue were completely forgotten; the sun was now shining in her heart.

When a log is put on the fire, the flames change what was cold, hard, and dense into heat and dancing light. This magic was seen by the sages as the gift of the official of the transformation of matter. In the body, the transformational fire is particularly strong in the small intestine, where the food we eat loses its form and identity and becomes part of us.

It is not only the food we eat that gets transformed. We ingest all our experiences, and the small intestine official must separate what is toxic or indigestible from what is a pure expression of love. There are many impurities to be eliminated, lest we become confused and tainted by the fear, greed, and aggression around us. For Adelle, the reliving of past pain and trauma showed that this official was burning out a poisonous past. The journey of transformation is always like this. With fierce compassion, fire destroys what needs to be destroyed. It doesn't stop its work to ask if we're comfortable with the process.

Some time ago, I was teaching at a place with a view of the chaparral, or miniature forest, across the border in Mexico a mile or two away. At one point, a wildfire broke out. Tall columns of flame lit up the night, and smoke blackened the sky during the day. No workers arrived to fight the blaze; no aircraft dumped water or chemicals. This fire continued for three or four days, and then it simply went out.

I was familiar with the chaparral; I had lived in it on the U.S. side of the border. To keep themselves from drying out during the hot, rainless summers, the plants coat themselves with waxes and oils, which build up year after year. Eventually a lightning strike starts a fire that burns to the edges of the volatile buildup. The fresher plants beyond are not very good fuel, so the fire goes out after it has burnt a few acres.

The burned area is invigorated. The soil has been enriched with minerals in the ash and now receives direct sunlight. There is the opportunity for new growth. In fact, some seeds will sprout only if they have been burned. The young plants are succulent and nutritious. They provide the best grazing for the many animals who come to feast and the best hunting for the humans who come looking for game. Within a couple of years, the forest has restored itself. The only evidence of the blaze is an area of particularly vigorous growth. The people understand that fire feeds a beneficial natural cycle of destruction and regeneration—at least, in Mexico they do.

In the United States, it would be unthinkable to let the chaparral burn. We distrust fire—that is to say, we distrust the Supreme Controller who looks after the world. We distrust natural cycles of destruction and transformation because those cycles cause losses, and we don't want to lose anything, even if the loss is beneficial. We try to control the natural world to avoid loss, so fire is suppressed. Like all human efforts to control the world, it brings on only more of what we were trying to avoid.

Instead of low, small brush fires keeping the forests fresh and vigorous, we now have vast areas becoming, year by year, drier and more volatile. When at last the match drops or the lightning strikes, we have conflagrations of tens of thousands of acres, producing enough heat to destroy ancient oaks and sycamores, enough to consume housing tracts, to melt automobiles.

The same holds true in our personal lives. Fire provokes small brushfires of conflict in our lives. This illuminates problem areas and prepares the way for resolution that leaves our inner landscape transformed and invigorated with new growth. But we fear these fires. We think conflict might cause us to lose something, be it affection, respect, or an opportunity for promotion. So we suppress the fire. We try to keep everything under control.

As years go by, the suppression causes more and more tinder to build up inside. That's why Adelle experienced quite a conflagration after the plant spirits gave her a spark. Earlier in this chapter, I quoted the letters of my student Charlotte, who wrote so expressively about what it was like for her to catch fire. Adelle and Charlotte are not unusual. Fire is suppressed throughout our society. There are vast amounts of volatile tinder out there. It's obvious what is to come.

In fact, huge wildfires are already burning: violence, war, political and economic strife, natural disasters. They will have to burn themselves out before humanity can get the tender, succulent new growth we need. Meanwhile, remember who controls the world, and trust the compassion that brings destruction and transformation.

QUESTIONS FIRE AND YOU

By answering these questions, you can savor and explore your relationship to the element of Fire. Relax for a moment by a flame—a candle flame would be fine. Enjoy the blaze, thank it for its presence, and invite it to shed light on your experiences. Consider these questions one by one, and address the answers to the fire itself. Feel free to laugh or cry. Say what is in your heart. Contradict yourself if you like. Honest answers are right answers.

1. When was the last time you had a really good laugh?

2. How do you feel in hot weather? Cold weather?

3. Do you go "hot and cold" about people? About things?

4. How do you feel about hot food? Hot music?

5. Do you wear red clothes? Would you buy a red car? Live in a red house?

6. How do you feel about summer?

7. What or whom do you feel passionate about?

8. What do you do for fun?

9. When have you felt heartbroken?

10. When have you felt disheartened?

11. When have you felt out of control?

12. When have you tried to control others?

13. Does your work bring you joy?

14. Does your family life bring you joy?

15. When have you felt vulnerable and unprotected?

16. How do you feel at parties?

17. Have you heard any good jokes lately?

18. How is your sex life?

19. What do you do wholeheartedly? Halfheartedly?

20. Do you enjoy being with people?

21. How important is friendship to you?

22. Do you perspire? Easily? With difficulty?

23. Do you have any circulatory problems?

24. How do you feel about being in the sun? Sunny weather? Cloudy weather?

25. When have you dreamed of fire or explosions?

26. Do you like bitter or burnt things, like coffee or burnt toast?

27. What do you feel bitter about?

28. Do you feel loved by your partner? Family? Friends? Associates?

29. When have you felt that you would never love again?

30. When have you felt your heart overflowing with love?

31. Do you know the people in your neighborhood?

32. Do you have a community you feel connected to?

33. Do you feel connected to nature?

34. Do you feel loved by nature?

35. How do you feel connected to God, Spirit, or the Divine?

36. Who do you love?

37. What do you love?

38. When have you isolated yourself?

39. How much time do you spend with live human beings? With electronic devices?

39. When have you been happy?

40. When have you felt peaceful joy?

41. Who are the wise elders in your life? How often do you speak to them?

42. What do you see burning in your life?

Which of these questions created the most feeling response in you? Which questions were difficult or easy to answer? Can you see where your fire, your passion for life, is strong or where it may be weak? Address the flame once again, and ask it for understanding that will help you perceive where the passion—the fire of your life—is almost gone, dying away, or wanting to blaze forth. Ask how and where you can burn more intensely and joyfully. Finally, sit quietly and allow yourself to feel both the joy and the heartache about what you see in your fire.

chapter 12

EARTH

Before I was born, my beautiful dark-brown Mother longed for me. She wanted to feel me suckling at her breast. She waited a long time for my arrival—many centuries, perhaps—until at last she could wait no longer. She removed two lumps of flesh from her own body and modeled them into a young woman and a young man. She made these young people beautiful in each other's eyes, and they joined together to bring forth a child, which was me. At last I had arrived! How happy my beautiful dark-brown Mother was! How contented!

Now that I had arrived, though, there was work to be done, for I was hungry and started crying for something to eat. My Mother caused the hairs of her beautiful dark-brown body to grow green and tall and to bear fruits and seeds. She made these foods beautiful and gave me eyes to feast on their beauty. She made them fragrant and gave me a nose to appreciate their perfume. She made them tasty and gave me a tongue to taste their exquisite flavors. She made them nutritious and gave me a stomach to digest their juices and turn my Mother's flesh into my own.

My beautiful dark-brown Mother knows that if I were to stray from her, I would soon become weak and emaciated. For this reason, she keeps me with her, always pressing her body against the soles of my feet. I feel her underneath me, and I know who I am and where I stand.

Because we are together constantly, I am learning from her example. She understands me, so I am learning how to understand others. She feeds me, so I am learning to feel secure and open handed. She has never abandoned me, so I have learned loyalty. She has never forgotten me, so I have learned how to remember. Perhaps memory is the greatest gift she has given me, because it is the only one I can give her in return.

This is your story, too. You and I have the same beautiful dark-brown Mother. Let us give the best thanks a grateful child can offer: "Beautiful dark-brown Mother, we remember you with love."

I am here thanks to many meals eaten by many people. The same could be said of my home, my family, this book, and the computer I am writing on. People and their accomplishments are made of food, and food is born of the soil. Earth is our Mother.

How well do we remember our Mother? Can we recall her ten thousand years of labor to create each inch of soil? Agricultural experts talk of "acceptable rates of erosion," while Midwestern dirt drifts down the Mississippi River. Have we forgotten who feeds us? Once we are all finally taken off her breast, who will bring us our food? Where will we get it?

A mother's breasts freely give her children nourishment, security, identity, and fulfillment. Our society hates mother's breasts and does everything it can to keep children away from them, for we have come to believe that nourishment, security, identity, and fulfillment should be purchased. Women are no longer solely devoted to motherhood; they are members of the work force, earning money to try to buy the things for their children that only their breasts can really provide.

In many less industrialized societies, mothers know that children need to nurse and to continue nursing, often for two, three, or even four years. In such cultures, breasts are openly displayed, without shame or provocation. Many of us in the United States, on the other hand, have never had our need for the breast fulfilled, and so it persists as an obsession in adult life. Our dissatisfaction and rage at not having enough of Mother distorts our fascination. We reject the real, serviceable, sagging maternal breast. It is the idealized virgin breast we crave. Thus we have created such modern inventions as the brassiere, the silicone implant, and breast cancer. Thus we have also rejected feminine values such as cooperation, nurturing, and sympathy. Thus we have substituted idealized, sterile foods for real ones. And thus, finally, we have the rape of Mother in all her forms, including soil, forests, wildlife, and the bodies of women.

From our first day to our last, we conduct an intimate relationship with Mother Earth through our mouths. As an organ of eating, our mouth is an extension of our stomach, and so our stomach keeps us connected to Mother Earth. Most people nowadays are aware that what goes into the stomach can either support health or tear it down. Are we also aware that the mind has a stomach that must be properly fed? How nutritious was your mental diet today? A well-filled stomach brings contentment, and a contented person is not envious, greedy, or competitive. A contented person does not feel superior or inferior and has no need to measure up to others. Contentment brings gratitude and the ability to sympathize. Did your mental diet bring you contentment today? Did you feed yourself on understanding and brotherhood or stress and violence?

These days everyone has a certain amount of stress and violence in their diet, but as long as we don't overindulge, a healthy stomach can churn it, mix it, and rot it down into digestible form. In the same way, the stomach gives us our ability to turn over an experience in our mind. In the West, we call this "rumination." In China, they say the stomach gives people the ability to ponder. If the stomach is weak, however, even bland food can be indigestible. Similarly, our mind can churn over innocuous experiences again and again in a vain effort to break them down and assimilate them; this churning is worry and, eventually, obsession.

The pondering, potentially obsessive, faculty of the stomach is beautifully expressed in Auguste Rodin's famous statue *The Thinker*. It is no coincidence that Rodin was a Frenchman, for the French are known to be stomach oriented. Witness their obsession with food—particularly food that has been worried over and rotted down, such as ripe cheeses, aged wines, and elaborate sauces. The French are constantly chewing something over, and if there is no food at hand, an idea will do just fine.

Whether in France or elsewhere, middle-class life offers many opportunities to feed the body and the mind. Physical food is never farther away than the corner convenience store, and with electronic media, we don't even have to leave our own homes to find food for the mind. But where do we go to find nourishment for our spirit? Are there convenience stores—or any stores at all—that provide food of this kind? The spirit has a stomach that needs to be fed regularly and well. A hungry spirit feels deprived and insecure. It may make an elaborate show of giving to others, but really there is nothing to give. A starving spirit eventually gives up the struggle and resigns itself to slow, wasting death.

Once an old man came to me for help. Since he could not walk, he had to be carried into my office. This was not difficult to do, for he weighed no more than sixty-five pounds in his soaking-wet diaper. He was placed on my couch. I took his cool hand and welcomed him, but he did not respond to my greeting and instead lay there staring at the wall. The nauseating, sweet odor of his body and the dirty-yellow color of his complexion made an interview unnecessary, though. Clearly his Earth element was impoverished.

I looked at this man sympathetically and asked him only one question: "Do you have an appetite?"

"No," he replied.

I brought him a plant spirit to strengthen the spirit of his stomach. Immediately he turned, looked me in the eye and said, "I could go for some good barbecue right now!"

After a little more chitchat, he was ready to leave. Although he moved very slowly and needed two people to help him, he insisted on walking. For the next hour, as I was treating other members of his family, I heard him in the waiting room, complaining loudly: "I'm starving! Let's get out of this place and go get us some barbecue!" At last his family took him to a nearby restaurant, where he ate a hearty portion.

Mothers need to be strong. As anyone who has tried it knows, mothering involves a lot of hard work. Within the body, the work of mothering is done by the spleen and pancreas, which transport nourishment from the stomach to the cells. It is as if they ran a shipping firm with thousands of yellow trucks delivering glucose to every part of the country. The spleen and pancreas function is dynamic and muscular and enables us to be dynamic and muscular as well. It is another of Mother Earth's gifts and another aspect of her genius; to every creature with a mouth, she gives muscles to get food.

This function of bringing the sugar to the cells or bringing the sweetness to life is a deceptively simple one. If modern life more often tastes bitter and metallic, it is because our spleen and/or pancreas is too ill to do its job. Symptoms of this illness are everywhere; the most obvious one is our addiction to sugar. It is worth noting that table sugar is a machine-made product. Industrial technology makes sugar refining possible, and it also creates the need for this addictive substance, because industrialized society produces people who do not know the sweetness of being supported by the earth. Such people are so deprived of sweetness that they will buy it regardless of the cost to their own health. In the world today, the universal artifact of our culture, more widely available than penicillin, gasoline, polyester, or rock and roll, is Coca-Cola.

Another symptom of our spleen/pancreas imbalance is our transportation network gone berserk. As we have seen, the function of a healthy transportation system is simply to deliver the goods and services necessary for the support of the people. In our society, however, transportation has become an end in itself. It has long since ceased to be our servant and has instead become our master, exacting heavy tribute through car payments, insurance, parking, garage construction, repair bills, gasoline prices, taxes to support road construction and maintenance, subsidies to transportation industries, and standing armies and military interventions designed to protect access to petroleum. If this weren't enough, our cancerous transportation system has made our air unfit to breathe and our water unfit to drink. It has given us a country where people suffer from ulcers, hypertension, and all manner of other diseases related to the stress of getting to work and back—a country where the noise and smell of the automobile penetrates every forest and meadow, a country where we don't know how to live without cars and trucks. This is so incredible that it bears repeating: *we no longer know how to live without cars and trucks!*

In most temples of transportation—auto-parts houses, repair shops, showrooms, truck stops, and dispatch offices—one usually finds a little shrine in which is displayed the image of a mythological sacred object. The object itself was lost long ago, and this primordial loss caused many people to dash madly about trying to find it. This dash was the birth of the modern transportation industry. No one has yet recovered this sacred object, but each man who takes up the search secretly believes he will be the chosen one. The sacred object, of course, is the female breast.

Carolina was a woman who helped my wife with the cooking and cleaning during the week. On weekends her pleasure was to walk to her plot of land in the hills outside of town and tend her corn. In late summer one year, the earth brought forth a bumper crop. Carolina saved her money and bought a small mare to pack in the harvest. A mare didn't need costly gasoline or repairs. Her wastes enriched rather than polluted the environment. She would eventually pay for herself with her foals. And there was no need to put pictures of tits on the mare because she came equipped with real ones of her own.

The Lakota shaman Wallace Black Elk was once asked by a sincere young man what we could do to heal the earth. He replied this way: "We don't have to heal the Earth; she can heal herself. All we have to do is stop making her sick." To this simple truth, I would add that the earth can heal *us,* too. Despite the neglect and the devastation we have heaped upon her, despite our illness and our ignorance, our Mother still loves her children. She has not turned her back on us yet; her breasts are still full of the milk of sympathy and understanding.

Robert, a physician in his mid-fifties, discovered a way to help his patients heal the pain of their minds and spirits as well as their physical complaints, and he initiated a program in one of the major hospitals in his area. His success aroused the envy and suspicion of his colleagues, who did not understand his work. Robert was subjected to humiliation by the hospital bureaucracy and was eventually fired. Around the same time, his wife divorced him and kicked him out of his home. Within a few months, he contracted a serious illness. His doctors diagnosed hepatitis and a large tumor, presumed malignant, in the neck of his pancreas. As a doctor, Robert knew such a cancer is untreatable and fatal, and in a whirlpool of fear and worry, he began to put his affairs in order. His scant strength was fading quickly, as he was unable to eat. Because he could not get up, he called me to his bedside.

Robert told me his story with desperate attention to detail. He clearly longed for me to understand, to know, and to fully sympathize with how he was feeling. His longing touched me and showed me his need for his Mother. I summoned Her in the form of a plant spirit and then got up to go. To my surprise, he leapt to his feet and followed me out the door of his bedroom. He proceeded directly to the kitchen, opened the refrigerator, and stood there grazing hungrily as I left the apartment. When I saw him again two weeks later, he was active and confident. Far from being bedridden, he was about to leave for Germany to visit a spiritual teacher who bills herself as an incarnation of the Divine Mother.

QUESTIONS EARTH AND YOU

When you are really hungry, take your favorite food to a pleasant place in nature. Give thanks and eat your food slowly. Note how it feels in your mouth and stomach. Pay attention also to how your surroundings make you feel. Then consider the questions below. Chew them, digest them, and answer them from your gut. By answering these questions, you can taste your relationship to the Earth element.

1. How do you feel about your mother?

2. How do you feel about your home?

3. What makes you feel secure? Insecure?

4. Do you feel that people understand you?

5. Are you able to nurture others?

6. How do you take care of yourself?

7. Do you care for others at your own expense?

8. How much do you worry?

9. Do you feel you are too fat? Too thin?

10. Do you overeat or eat when you are not hungry? If so, why?

11. Do you eat foods that really satisfy you?

12. Do you enjoy eating?

13. If you are a woman, how do you feel about your breasts? If you are a man, how do you feel about women's breasts?

14. Were you breastfed? If so, for how long? How do you feel when you watch a child being breastfed?

15. Do you enjoy sweets?

16. How is your digestion?

17. What makes you nauseated? What makes you vomit?

18. How do you feel about walking barefooted? Putting your hands in dirt?

19. Would you like to be alone in the wilderness?

20. How do you feel about caring for young children?

21. Would you paint your kitchen yellow? Your living room? Your car?

22. How do you feel in Indian summer (harvest time)?

23. When have you felt that the rug was pulled out from under you?

24. What makes you feel grounded? Ungrounded?

25. What obsessions do you have?

26. How is your memory?

27. Do you have a shoulder to cry on? A sympathetic ear to listen to your problems?

28. How do you know who you are?

29. Do you know where your next meal is coming from?

30. Are you a sympathetic listener?

31. Do you know how people feel? Do you care how they feel?

32. How do you feel when a homeless person asks you for money?

33. Do you enjoy taking care of people? Animals?

34. Plants, rocks, rivers, wind, mountains, valleys—do you know how they feel? Do their feelings matter to you?

35. What do you feel grateful for today?

Earth gives the nourishment and support we need. As you consider your answers to these questions, see how the natural world and people (including yourself) support you. What were the issues in which your insecurities clustered? What gives you the greatest stability? Go outside and sit on the ground and feel the earth giving you the support and nourishment you need in your life today. Feel your body relax and your mind grow calm. Both your security and insecurity bring you close to the one who feeds your flesh, your mind, and your soul: Mother Earth.

chapter 13

METAL

The old shaman, don Guadalupe González Ríos, led us on a spiritual pilgrimage to the holy land where his gods dwell. We fasted in preparation and went to a sacred spring, where the old man anointed us with holy water. After that, he guided us into the wilderness, where we confessed, telling Grandfather Fire the name of every sexual partner we ever had. Only then were we pure enough to receive the blessings we sought.

After we entered the hallowed valley, don Guadalupe built an altar under the open sky. On a whoosh of Hawk's wing, he passed each of us as much spiritual power as we had the strength to withstand. He lit and blessed a fire and brought us around it. Then he sat and watched over us as the secret essence did its work.

Many hours passed. Night fell. The moon rose and was sung to by the coyotes. We were still in a circle around the fire under the starlit sky. Sensing we were now settled enough to receive his words, the old shaman spoke:

"You have traveled a long way and made a lot of sacrifice to come here, to receive something. I have put my secret into you so you won't say, 'I went to see the great shaman so-and-so, and he didn't give me anything.' No, I'm not like some who deny what they know because they don't want to share it. I am going to die some day. What is the use of having learned something if I can't pass it on? I would like everyone to be able to know what I know!

"I want you people to understand that everything I have, I owe to my father. When I was very little, maybe three or four years old, my father carried me on his back up the holy mountain where the Wind Tree lives. When we got to the summit, he lit candles and left offerings for me. He stayed up all night praying for me. I didn't know what was going on; I just fell asleep. Years later, when he asked me if I remembered those journeys, I told him I didn't. He said, 'Of course not! You were asleep most of the time!'

"When I got a little older my father called me to his side and said, 'Listen, my son. I am just a poor Indian. When I die you will not inherit cattle, you will not inherit a house or money. But you will inherit a path of healing and knowledge, a way through life that will sustain you.' I told my father that it was good, that I accepted his gift. 'I am going to give you my heart,' he said. 'You will inherit my heart.' And he put his secret into me.

"From the time I was twelve years old, I didn't bother my father any more; on my own I started making pilgrimages to the mountain. I went every year for six years, and then I maintained my vows for another six. Then I came for six years to this place where we are now sitting, and I maintained my vows for six years after that. By the time I was four or five years into my apprenticeship, I saw that what my father had said was coming to pass. The deer would come and offer themselves to me. And those who came to be touched by my hand were healed and made well. It was just as he had said it would be.

"At one point I wandered off the path my father had given me. I began looking for a different life. But it went badly for me, and I returned. Forty-eight years and more I have been walking this path of knowledge and healing, and it supports me to this day.

"There have been times when I doubted that my father was even my father. But I know he was my father: he planted the seed of wisdom in me. I owe everything to him. I thank God for my father!

"That is all I want to say to you. Now you know a little bit about the traditions of my people. You speak to me now. Tell me about your traditions."

"Don Guadalupe," I said, "My people have lost our traditions."

"How can this be?" he asked. "The spiritual tradition is fundamental. It is the first thing a person should have."

"With no one to guide us," I replied, "we cannot find the way. That is why we have come from so far to be here with you. None of us had a father like yours to teach us."

"No! Really?" asked the old man.

Betty turned to me, tears glistening in her eyes, and said, "Tell don Lupe this: Yesterday you told me to confess my partners to Grandfather Fire. I want you to know that the first name on my list was that of my father."

The shaman was stunned by this message. "With his own daughter? Like an animal? How can this be?"

"This is what my people have come to," I told him.

A father is the one who shows us the way through the world; through him, we come to know what is of value in life. His hand on our shoulder gives us the feeling of dignity and self-worth. He is the first and greatest authority. Because he respects us, we respect ourselves; because we respect ourselves, we respect others. The father's role is to recognize our essence, to encourage and instruct us so that it may come forth and bless our life with its unique quality.

Did your father do all that? If so, you are extremely fortunate; your life is rich, and your connection to spirit is strong. For you, every mundane experience is important and charged with significance.

Or was your father more like Betty's? He may not have violated your body, but perhaps he violated your soul with neglect. If so, you have suffered great loss, and your soul knows depths of grief.

Many of us go around dazed by unspent grief, looking for something to fill the hollow place in our chest. We seek the presence of the Father—our Father who art in heaven. He is the source of spiritual wealth, and if we can't find Him, we start looking for substitutes. Often we feel that material wealth will take His place. I need not document how corrosive to the soul this substitution can be. The Huichol Indian don Guadalupe was as shocked at the poverty of our people as we were at the poverty of his.

Some of us who lack our Father try to compensate by accumulating a wealth of information, facts, or learning. Don Guadalupe, who was illiterate, had no book learning to enrich him. He healed people and gave them strength by sharing his spiritual wealth. He did not share it through lecture, because spirit cannot be captured in words. He called his treasure his "secret." His sharing was a direct act of generosity from one soul to another.

Don Guadalupe used to show a lot of interest in the healing practices of medical doctors. One time, after a particularly profound session of instruction, he expressed satisfaction at my progress. Then he surprised me by asking if I thought a Huichol person would be capable of becoming a medical doctor.

"Of course," I replied. Trying to convey that Western medicine requires only a strong intellect, I said, "All that is needed to become a medical doctor is the ability to read very well." Since reading was a mystery to this man, my answer was not at all illuminating. I tried again. "That is to say, don Guadalupe, that in our medicine there is no secret."

"Ah!" he said. That was the last time I heard him express interest in the subject.

Another way to look for the Father is by accumulating supposed spiritual wealth. Here we find the desperate spiritual seekers who measure their worth by their importance in the sect of their choice, be it religion, therapy, art, science, politics, or even a corporation, police force, or the military. But the collectors of spiritual accolades, like the collectors of knowledge and the collectors of material wealth, don't realize that the Father is not limited to a particular temple. There is nothing special that needs to be accomplished in order to come into His presence. All you have to do is breathe. The Heavenly Father pervades the air around us and enters us through our lungs with every breath.

The essence of the Father is subtle, yet the ancient Chinese referred to it as Metal, the densest of the elements. Perhaps this is because metal is the most refined and valuable essence of the earth. In any case, people from many cultures have long accepted metals such as gold and silver as tokens of value. At some point in our history, we began to mistake the tokens for the real thing. The result has been centuries of slaughter and exploitation. The lust for a shiny yellow metal drove European people to come to America, massacre its peoples, and destroy the natural environment. They were able to do so thanks to knowledge of steel and with the blessings of a religion that worships God the Father. Lust for gold, allegiance to steel, violence to the spirit, and the cult of a ruthless god: these are the founding values of our Western nations.

Authority and power are at the core of the masculine principle in men and women alike, yet most of us do not know the difference between authority and suppression, between power and abuse. When was the last time you saw a judge, a police officer, a professor, or your own boss weep while on duty? When did we have a national day of mourning for the people we killed in Iraq, Vietnam, Hiroshima, or anyplace else?

Only recently did the men's movement discover that grief is the key to manhood. This came as a big surprise to many, because grief takes the cutting edge off strength and tempers it with kindness. But when we have been softened and made kind, we are more authentic, more powerful, and, ultimately, more authoritative.

Grief gets our values straight. It teaches respect. If grief has been deeply felt, a person who has just lost a loved one is clear about what is important and about how precious human life is. Our main problem with grief is that we don't like to feel it. We think we have to be strong in the conventional masculine sense instead.

This type of strength is not really strength at all, but rather a pathological refusal to let go. Before the essence of the Father can inspire us through our lungs, we must be clean, pure, and empty inside. This cleanliness is maintained by the colon, which removes filth and brings sparkle, righteousness, and receptivity to the body, mind, and spirit. There is an old Zen story that could be used to illustrate how the colon and lungs work together. This is my version of that story:

There once lived a prosperous merchant and his younger brother. The merchant had a successful business, a large family, and a reputation for righteousness. The brother, on the other hand, was a bachelor and a drifter who had never pursued any occupation for long. The merchant was astonished when his brother appeared one day and announced that he had married and that his wife was with child. He wanted employment, he said, in order to support his new family, and he begged the older brother to give him even the humblest position in his firm.

The merchant was impressed by his sincerity and eagerness, and he gladly gave him a job. He was at a loss to account for the sudden transformation in his brother, however, so he questioned him about it.

"Dear brother," the younger man replied, "all my life I have been driven by a desire to know the highest, the most sublime. Agriculture seemed trivial to me, and I was oppressed by the very thought of entering one of the trades or professions. I drifted about, looking for something of value, but my search was in vain, and life seemed pointless and depressing. At length I heard of an elderly man known as Grandfather. He was said to be a man of great wisdom, perhaps even a divine sage. In desperation I decided to go to him to ask for initiation into his cult."

"Yes, I have heard of this man," said the merchant. "Did you visit him? How did he receive you?"

"Indeed, I did visit him," said the younger man. "He was practicing the movements of tai chi when I arrived. He was as energetic as a man of middle years, despite his great age. After finishing his exercise, he greeted me with kindness and asked me the purpose of my visit.

"'After years of wandering and searching, I have found nothing of value,' I told him. 'Emptiness and sorrow are my lot. I have been told that you possess a great treasure of wisdom, and indeed the sparkle in your eyes and the serenity of your face testify that you have attained something that eludes me still. I have come to request that you teach me.'

"The old man told me, 'It is good that you have come, but I am looking for a disciple who knows how to be receptive. The master, you see, is active, and pours his wisdom into the disciple. It is rather like pouring a cup of tea. Truly your cup is empty and in need of filling. Unfortunately,' he said with a chuckle, 'you have not learned to hold your cup still. If I tried to teach you, my tea would end up being spilled on the table.'

"The interview seemed to have concluded, so I thanked him and took my leave. The old man's words were not lost on me. It was quite true! My quest had led me from one door to the next. I had never stayed with anything very long. No wonder I had been restless and unfulfilled! I decided to change my ways. I married, and I intend to stay here in this town, with your help, dear brother."

As years passed, the younger brother worked hard and became a partner in the firm. He seemed to grow ever more ingenious and productive as he prospered. He became a prominent civic leader and one of the most respected figures in his community.

Meanwhile, the other brother was not faring so well. His business still flourished, it is true, but he begrudged his younger brother his high status. Gradually the older man began to doubt himself. He became listless, and his health deteriorated. It happened that he heard of the elderly sage again, and now he resolved to visit him and ask for help. The master had refused to pour his blessings into his brother's teacup because he had been a weak and irresolute young man, but the older brother reasoned that he himself would be a worthy recipient of the choicest blessings because he had been strong and hard working all his life. Therefore, he thought, by approaching Grandfather he could find relief from suffering and show up his younger brother all in one stroke.

He journeyed to the abode of the sage and was greeted with warmth. The master said he had heard of the merchant's reputation and considered himself honored to entertain him. When the merchant explained that he had come to receive teachings, the master seemed very pleased indeed. The sage invited the merchant into his quarters and asked him to share a cup of tea.

"Aha!" thought the merchant. "The symbolic pouring of tea! Just as I thought! I indeed am a worthy disciple! Truly I know how to be receptive, for now the teacher is going to pour his inspiration into me."

The two were seated, and the tea set was brought. The host graciously lifted the teapot and began to pour into the cup of his guest, who looked on with a smile of self-congratulations. That smile faded into a look of consternation and then horror as the sage continued to pour. The tea reached the brim of the cup and began spilling onto the table. The host continued smiling and pouring. The puddle of tea on the tabletop widened. When the tea began to run onto the old man's clothing, it became clear that this so-called sage was an impostor, a soft-headed old lout who could not even pour a cup of tea, let alone confer blessings on others. The merchant could contain himself no longer. "Stop, you fool, stop!" he shouted. "Can't you see that my cup is full?"

"Ah," said the sage. "Your cup is so full. 'I am a great man. I am so clever. I am more worthy than my brother.' How can I pour anything into your cup? It is too full. Your brother's cup was empty when he came to me, and he received total enlightenment three years ago. *Empty your cup.*"

These words dazed and confounded the merchant. All thoughts and opinions were erased, and he became empty. In that state, he was truly a worthy disciple. What more can be said of the wordless moment when a man receives the spirit?

The merchant stayed on and studied under the sage for nine years. At the end of that time, he too attained enlightenment.

Pauline was a well-educated entrepreneur of forty years of age. Like most of those who come for help, she started out by telling me her physical problems: "I used to do massage, but my hands started hurting terribly. I went to the doctor, who said I had tendonitis. I stopped doing massage, but I got worse anyway. My hands got weak, no strength in them at all, and the pain was intense. My back started hurting too. A second doctor diagnosed carpal tunnel syndrome, and a third said I had two twisted cervical vertebrae. I took anti-inflammatories and also some natural therapies. I can do whatever I need to do now, but there is still a lot of tension, and it's a real effort to stand up straight.

"I'm having massages done myself now, and for three days after each one, I get fever, chills, and fatigue. Then I also get headaches and infections that go into my lungs. I keep having the taste of tobacco in my mouth, even though I quit smoking two years ago. And I still have a cough like the one I had when I had bronchitis years ago. Also, my trunk aches, as well as my left wrist and my left knee. If that weren't enough, my bowels are terrible too. I only go once a week."

I drew Pauline out about how she felt in herself: "Sometimes my spirits really aren't that great. I got married a few months ago, and my husband aggravates me. He contradicts me all the time. What a drag! I get kind of depressed. In fact, for the past week I have had zero energy, zero oomph. I'm just exhausted from constantly trying to get going. All the therapies, the massage—I just feel like giving up. It gets so bad that sometimes I don't want to go on living."

Responding to my question about her childhood, she said, "When I was little, I was the apple of my father's eye, but when I was four there was a total break with him, a total rupture. From that time on, the only time he said anything to me was to give me a bawling out for something or other. From thirteen on, I became very rebellious. I know now that I was trying to get some attention from him.

"What happened to cause the rupture with my father? I don't know for sure. I went for hypnosis to try and find out. A memory started coming back. It was vague, but I think there might have been something sexual with him. As soon as this started to come up, these incredible sobs started coming out of me. I cried and cried. Then I blocked the whole thing out, and that is all I know about it."

With Pauline, the white color of her complexion, the weeping tone of her voice, the slightly rotten odor of her body, and the predominant emotion of grief let me know that her suffering was caused by a severed connection with the Heavenly Father. With that understanding, her whole story made sense: the rupture with her physical father plunged the young Pauline into grief that stayed with her, unplumbed, for decades. When she came close to recalling the event as an adult under hypnosis, she wept uncontrollably but did not have the emotional strength to confront it directly. At puberty, she started acting out her lack of Father by rebelling against all forms of authority—that is to say, all forms of fathering. Meanwhile, the lack of inspiration from the heavens was slowly making her weaker, resulting in chronic lung problems, chronic colon problems, chronic pain, and exhaustion. Only at age forty did she come out of her rebellion enough to marry, and the man she chose was hypercritical, just as her father had been. This was the crisis for Pauline. Her pain now went so deep that she no longer wanted to live. At this moment, she was ready to find help.

Help came in the form of a plant spirit that led her back to her Heavenly Father. A week after her first treatment, Pauline's words were "I feel better. I feel strong, and I have hope." With that hope and that strength, Pauline started on the road back to life.

QUESTIONS METAL AND YOU

Wake up early in the morning, move your bowels, and go to the summit of a hill or mountain. Breathe deeply. Bow, kneel, or perform a solemn ceremony as a gesture of respect to the experiences of your own life. Take up these questions. Consider each answer to be a gem of priceless wisdom. By answering these questions, you can honor your relationship to Metal.

1. How do you feel about your father?

2. How do you feel in autumn?

3. When was the last time you wept?

4. When have you lost someone who was precious to you?

5. When have you lost valuable objects?

6. What golden opportunities have you lost?

7. What do you regret?

8. How are your bowels?

9. What grudges have you held?

10. How important is fresh, clean air to you?

11. Do you feel rich or poor? Why?

12. You have a chance to make a lot of money doing a job you don't believe in. Do you take it? Why?

13. What traditions do you observe? What traditions do you avoid observing? Why?

14. How do you feel around policemen? Bosses? Other authority figures?

15. Does your family respect you? Do your working companions respect you? Do you respect them?

16. What do you do to gain respect?

17. Do others admire you? How do you feel when they tell you they do?

18. Whom do you admire? Why?

19. How do you feel at funerals?

20. How do you feel when you make a mistake?

21. When was the last time you admitted making a mistake?

22. Do you like pungent, spicy foods?

23. Are you an authority on something? Do you enjoy being an authority?

24. Whose authority do you respect?

25. What do you collect?

26. How do you feel wearing white clothes?

27. What are you a purist about?

28. What are your strengths? Your weaknesses?

29. How much metal do you wear?

30. How do you feel around strong men? Weak men?

31. What is your religion or spiritual path?

32. What or whom do you honor?

33. When have you done something dishonorable?

34. What is the most precious thing in your life?

The energy of Father in all forms of life can wound us, challenge us, or anger us. What leads us, sharpens our lives, brings authority and guidance, or gives us riches are mixed together to give us the gains and losses of our life. What in these questions depresses and saddens you? Where in you are the hidden, metallic, steel-like strengths that you need to grow and expand? Go outdoors and breathe deeply. Breath is the source of power that connects us to the Father. Ask this metallic, heavenly power to strengthen and firm your life, to heal loss, welcome opportunity, and gain new capability to act and live in the world. Sit now in the center of these feelings and insights and be respectful to the one who breathes life into your body, mind, and spirit: your Heavenly Father.

chapter 14

WATER

On the summit of a mountain in central Mexico stands a small pyramid known as El Tepozteco. When I first visited it, this monument captured my imagination. What was it used for, I wondered; what gods were honored here? I asked friends about it, but they were almost as ignorant as I was. I was told only that the structure was dedicated to two deities: Quetzalcoatl and Tlaloc. These names meant nothing to me, so I determined to find out about the pyramid for myself. I climbed the mountain, scaled the walls, and lay down on the ceremonial platform with some apprehension. Did I have the right to be here without a guide? Was I being disrespectful? Was this where priests with obsidian knives cut the still-beating hearts out of their human victims? Or was it the Incas in Peru who did that? I closed my eyes and hoped for the best.

A jaguar appears. He circles quickly around the pyramid, his tail held straight up. Suddenly he wheels and faces me. "So," he says, "you want to meet Tlaloc, eh?"

"Well, yes, I suppose I would like to meet him," I reply. "How do I do that?"

"I'll take you. Get on my back."

I mount the jaguar. He leaps into the air and bounds upward. We reach the sky and tear through it as if it were a paper screen. We find ourselves in another, more colorful world under a different sky. The cat continues upward. He tears through this new sky, and we enter a third world. He keeps running, tearing through sky after sky.

In the thirteenth world, the jaguar comes to a halt and tells me to dismount. As I do so, I look over the edge of the small plain where I find myself. Below me I see the worlds I have just passed through, neatly stacked like the steps of the pyramid.

Turning around, I see a young man with long blond hair, blue eyes, and a halo. His palms are facing forward, and from the center of each palm spurts a stream of water. These streams flow down through the worlds below, eventually forming the waters of our earth, where fish swim and plants flourish.

The young man speaks. "Hello! I'm Tlaloc!"

"You are Tlaloc?"

"Yes."

"Then how come you have blond hair and blue eyes?"

"You see me as a gringo because you are a gringo. The people who built this pyramid saw me differently. I look different to different folks, but everyone knows me. I am the Rain God."

"It is a privilege to meet you. Please tell me something about yourself."

"You are a student and doctor of the elements," says Tlaloc. "Tell me what you know about rain, about water."

"Have you got a minute?" I ask.

"Sure," replies the deity, taking a seat and lighting a cigarette.

"Okay, here goes—water is sacred and mysterious, the origin of life. I've often wondered why life chose to take birth in the sea. I think the answer is in how responsive water is. The first thing about living creatures is that they move and are still by turns, and water is the element that supports movement and stillness alike. There are so many movements: our joints move in water, our food is digested in water, our sperm swims in water, our brains think in water. The surging of water causes the movements of our souls: the willpower, the ambition. And there is stillness, too. When the water in us comes to rest, we know peace and plunge

118

beneath the surface of appearances. There are eternal moments between breaths, between thoughts."

Suddenly I feel timid giving a lecture to a god. "How am I doing?" I ask.

"Fine!" says Tlaloc, "Keep going."

"Well, the only other thing I want to mention is death. Every living thing seeks life and fears death, so water is both the source of life and the source of fear as well as awe, which is a sublime form of fear."

"That was very good!" Tlaloc says. "You should be telling people these things! People need to know the things you just said, and more. There is more to say."

"Like what?" I ask.

"Look at the way people squander water. Look how they pollute it. They don't realize they are utterly dependent on rainfall, that water is the very blood in their veins. For most people, water is just a commodity to be bought and sold; something that comes out of a faucet. To them, rain is a nuisance that makes driving inconvenient. They treat me as if I had no feelings. Naturally, I treat them the same way. Diseases, phobias, exhaustion, floods, droughts—what do they expect?"

"And you want me to tell people about this?"

"Yes, tell them. They need to know."

"They won't believe me! I'm not even sure I believe me! Am I actually having this conversation, or am I making it up?"

"You will see," says Tlaloc. "After a while, you will get a sign, a coincidence. This will convince you I am for real. Meanwhile, it has been very nice meeting with you. You may go now."

I thank Tlaloc and ask the jaguar to return me to my world.

Several months later, I visited my sister in California. On her bookshelf, a certain volume caught my eye: *Mesoamerican Mythology.* I took the book down and opened it at random. There was a photograph of an Aztec bas-relief. At the top of the carving stood a young man with his hands at his sides, palms facing forward. A stream of water spurted from each palm and flowed into the world below, where fish swam and plants flourished on riverbanks. The caption read: "Tlaloc, Aztec Rain God." Here was the coincidence I had been promised!

I considered the words of the deity: "They treat me as if I had no feelings." It was true. My patients were polluting their inner waters with all manner of toxic substances. They were using stimulants; they were overworking, depleting their reservoirs of ambition and will, and then they were coming to me with the resultant symptoms: depression, anxiety, fatigue, phobias, arthritis. On a larger scale, we were treating the waters of the earth the same way—polluting them with pesticides, herbicides, heavy metals, nuclear wastes, and God knows what else. In my own town, local officials were pumping more water out of the ground than rainfall could replenish.

It wasn't always this way for humankind. There was a time—a long, long time—when we knew we are related to Water.

When my sister-in-law went to visit the Tarahumara Indians in Mexico, they were having a serious drought. Their crops, and therefore their lives, were in danger, so the community got together under the guidance of the shamans. They sang and danced to the rain god all night. At sunrise a thunderstorm drenched the happy dancers.

We can scarcely imagine the communion those Indians must have enjoyed. We may not even believe such a thing is possible, so alienated from Water have we become. Yet this kind of interaction with Water used to be the norm for all humanity. This was how we survived until just yesterday.

It is still possible today. After I met Tlaloc, I made a dream journey to ask for help for the drought we were having. He gave me a ceremony for bringing rain. It required certain props, including a picture of Tlaloc drawn by me and candles made of chocolate. I drew an awkward little cartoon and set about making the candles. The first one turned out well enough to keep a small flame going. After lighting it, I absent-mindedly set it down in front of the cartoon. Within fourteen hours, an unpredicted storm rolled in and blessed the town with rain. That storm was followed by several others.

There was no need to call on Tlaloc again until the following year, which was also dry. I performed the full ceremony for the first time on February 3, 1987, in Santa Barbara, California. It was a hot day with clear skies. No rain had fallen and none was forecast, but when I awoke the following morning there were tiny craters in the dust. A few raindrops had fallen during the night. The following days were sunny and dry, though, and it seemed to me the ceremony had failed.

I visited the rain god again on February 8. "What went wrong with the ceremony?" I asked.

"Nothing. I thought it was charming," he replied. "I sent you a sprinkle to let you know you did a good job."

"Is there something more I can do so we can get enough rain this year?"

Tlaloc frowned. "If people get enough rain every year, they take it for granted. They don't learn anything that way."

"But you don't want nature to suffer, do you?" I asked.

"The plants and animals will survive a year of drought and fire. You should be talking to people and telling them what you know rather than wasting your time here with me."

"I don't know if I can do that," I said. "I don't have the confidence. If I don't get another good synchronicity, I'm going to doubt this whole thing again. You've got to send me some serious rain."

"Can you give me another candle?" asked Tlaloc.

"Sure."

"Okay then, you've got a deal."

I lit a chocolate candle and sat down to compose an article about the rain god. If he was for real, it would rain, and I would have to tell people what I knew. If it didn't rain, I wouldn't bother to finish the composition.

I started to write at three in the afternoon. A wind came up and clouds thickened. At five-thirty, it rained for a few seconds. After midnight, it started to come down hard and steady. I finished my article and promised Tlaloc I would begin teaching.

A few years later I was living in the Sierra Foothills of Northern California. The country was in the second year of disastrous drought. The previous year I had read a newspaper article about a group of Iowa farmers who pooled their money and hired a Lakota shaman and his troupe of rain dancers from the Rosebud Reservation in South Dakota. The Indians arrived and performed their ceremony. It rained three days later, as promised. If this could happen in Iowa, it could happen anywhere, I reasoned, because farmers everywhere are practical people. Now was the time to demonstrate a practical alternative to treating water as if it had no feelings. I would offer rainmaking services to ranchers and farmers. If I was successful, they would pay a fee and agree to make certain changes that would put them on better terms with water. If I was not successful, there would be no charge or obligation.

I presented my scheme to the rain god. I told him I didn't have the credentials of a Native American medicine man. Before anyone would take me seriously, I needed to produce some undeniable results. I asked him to send enough rain to keep the grass green in my yard throughout the summer—a miracle in that part of the country. He agreed to help but set two conditions. First, I had to understand that this project was only for helping people find a better way to live. It was not to be my personal ego trip. Second, I had to declare my intention in public before we started; if I wasn't willing to risk ridicule, I might as well forget the whole thing. I agreed to his conditions. I took out ads in the local newspapers announcing my project and started performing his ceremony regularly.

It continued to rain through the spring and into the summer. By mid-July, the grass was still green under the oaks in my back yard. Meanwhile, crops and livestock were perishing of thirst in the Midwest and Southwest. I felt the time had come to reach out. I renewed contact with Allan Savory of the Center for Holistic Management—now called Holistic Management International—in Albuquerque (holisticmanagement.org). Allan teaches brilliant, unorthodox agricultural management methods. Because his clients are among the world's most open-minded farmers, I asked Allan to present my offer to them.

Allan explained that the major obstacle he faces in his work is public acceptance. If he went around talking about rainmaking, folks would think for sure he was crazy, so he had to decline to present my offer. Two weeks later, though, he thought again. He was giving a seminar in the hardest-hit part of Texas. The ranchers were telling tales of cracked earth, dying cattle, and bankruptcy. "Here," he thought to himself, "is a group that has nothing to lose and everything to gain." He presented my rainmaking offer. Not a single person responded or even acknowledged that the offer had been made. They all went on talking as if nothing had happened.

The Tlaloc project was to be for the benefit of others, but nobody was ready to benefit from it, so I stopped performing the ceremony. It stopped raining. The grass in my yard turned brown. I was not able to help anyone else, but at least I convinced myself that there is a rain god who treats us the way we treat him.

We have to meet every moment with the right juices. Danger needs adrenaline, food needs digestive fluid, sex calls for other fluids. Everything juicy is water and is pooled by the bladder spirit. Even our energy flows as a fluid and pools there. When the pool is full, we flow with the changes like water does. If the pool runs dry, there is fear, paralysis—no flow.

The kidney spirit harbors deep mysteries of water. Consider winter, the season of water. A seed sleeps, gestating under the snow in the dark stillness of the earth-womb. Deep within itself it finds the primeval chaos giving birth to the world. It has arrived at the life spring. Drinking here, the seed imbibes the will to live. Its waters have been charged with a force that brings life out of death and being out of nothingness. It will carry this force into the world, and it will pass a drop of it through its sexual fluids into its own seeds.

This force, which is harbored by the kidneys, cannot be adequately described; we can only point to some of its effects. The Chinese sages said the kidney is the origin and basis of the life force. A Middle Eastern sage said, "Unless you are born of water and the spirit, you cannot enter the Kingdom of God."

Plants do not have kidneys or bladders, but they store fluids and harbor the mysterious life spring just as we do. What is more, they will bring peace to our waters if we ask them to.

Roberta, a woman in her mid-thirties, is an example of someone who benefited from plant spirits' power with water. As I listened to Roberta's complaints during her first visit, I heard the groaning sound of her voice, saw the blue color of her complexion, smelled the putrid aroma of a stagnant pond, sensed the fear that had paralyzed her, and noticed the theme of water imbalance repeat itself in her life story:

I used to sleep fourteen hours a night, but I can't sleep at all now unless I get a massage. I feel very bad, defeated; I can't go on. There is a hole in my stomach. I have no inner peace, just constant anxiety.

When I was a girl, I was in bed for three years with nephritis, a kidney disease. By the time I was twelve, I was living in a total fantasy world. I would lie in my sickbed and masturbate hour after hour. It wasn't so much for the pleasure of it; I was just trying to escape from anxiety. But anyway, my sexuality got out of control. I've had about eight abortions, I guess. I've lost count. But I feel very guilty about that and afraid of the consequences.

I've always been one to drift with the tides. My boyfriend of the moment always directed things. After I broke up with somebody in Spain, I was so depressed I couldn't get out of bed. This healer finally got me up, and I went to work. I made tons and tons of money, but I pissed it all away. Like I say, I just drift with the tides.

My mother was very possessive, very critical. She was perfect and always pointed out my imperfections. My father just died three months ago, and that's when I really lost it. He was almost God to me—a brilliant painter, poet, philosopher. On the other hand, he scared the pee out of me too. He was very violent; he used to beat me with his belt. I've lived my whole life in terror of him. And come to think of it, I've been prone to trembling ever since I was a little girl.

Now I feel as if I have run out of water. Everything is dry. It's as if my life is a landscape of salt.

I called on a plant spirit to bring the waters of life back to Roberta. At her second visit, she said she was feeling well in the daytime and wanting to be active again. At night she was sleeping more but was bothered by nightmares of fish. By her third visit, she had entered a kind of winter-time hibernation. She was spending her days dreaming and musing in her darkened bedroom. Roberta never showed up for her fourth visit. She was out looking for a job.

If you think Roberta's story of a life lived in anxiety and escapist fantasy is shocking and sad, I agree with you. If you think her condition is rare, I'm not sure I would agree.

There is a less polite synonym for anxiety: *fear.* Nervousness is also fear. Concern is a form of fear. Most stress is fear. Tension is caused by fear. Worry is based in fear. To be emotionally numb betrays a fear of feeling. Even thinking is a fearful way of trying to avoid fear.

Who these days can claim their life is free from anxiety, nervousness, concern, stress, tension, worry, numbness, or thinking? How many people engage in escapist strategies such as television, movies, computer games, reading, spectator sports, overeating, drugs, alcohol, dysfunctional love affairs, pornography, overexertion, shopping, and so on? Let's have a square look at this unpopular subject. What is fear? What is its role? What does it provide?

First of all, fear is an emotion. Like other emotions, fear is natural. It has a legitimate role. It protects our life by giving us what we need to flee from danger or overcome it. This the famous fight-or-flight response, produced by adrenaline, which is secreted by a gland attached to the kidneys. By fueling this response, fear gives us the extra boost we need to jump out of the way of the oncoming bus or the strength to fight off an attacker. At this level, where clear and present danger is responded to without thought, fear is necessary and good.

The next level is where our mind identifies danger and comes up with a scheme to control the situation and create a "good" outcome. In the old days, such situations played out something like this: "I am hungry; my family is too. We could all starve. There are plenty of deer in these woods, but they are faster and more nimble than I. I have a clever plan, though. I'll fasten this sharp stone to that straight stick with some plant fibers. Then I'll throw the thing at the next deer I see, and we will have a meal."

There was a twentieth-century version of this old story in horror films. A seemingly invincible monster threatens a desirable young woman—and the rest of the world, by the way. A brainy young scientist comes up with a clever plan, kills the monster, and saves the girl, who adoringly falls into his arms. Incidentally, the rest of the world is saved too.

Fear, with its clever plans, has killed many deer, but it cannot really slay the monster, because the monster is fear itself. Actions driven by fear will always produce more fear. In the old days, it was simple. After feasting on the deer, the family eventually got hungry again. The concern drove another hunt. It was not expected that fear would be banished forever. Fear was accepted as part of life. It came and it went, and that was okay.

Somewhere along the way, though, people got overly impressed with the successes of the mind. Its strategies seemed so effective at controlling things! Life became a game of control in order to banish the fear of losing something. The strategy was to get more for yourself—more grain, more land, more cattle, more natural resources, more slaves, more women, more money, more power, more fame, more hostile corporate takeovers, more everything. Greed tried to outrun the monster. But the more you have, the more you fear losing, so the monster lives on, chasing you to your grave. Along the way, you forget you are part of a miraculous natural world designed to give you what you need.

Our society feeds and reinforces fear. The clever strategies of the mind are held as the highest value. We are dazzled by their false promises and blind to the hamster wheel that powers them. The mind, thus lionized, usurps the throne of the Supreme Controller. Like all dictators, it wants more and more control of its own. From that perch, the emotions, unruly as they can be, are seen as dangerous. Instead of being allowed to flow as they will, the emotions are dammed up. Behind the dam of fear, they grow ever bigger and more forceful. Fear, which was designed to protect us from danger, has now itself become a danger. Groaning and shuddering with the strain, the dam finally bursts. We will do almost anything to save ourselves from the flood; we don't stop to consider consequences.

Does life seem like a tsunami? Like a parched desert? Could it be that we have ignored the feelings of the rain god? Have we spurned his gifts? Plant spirit medicine helps bring down the dams. It opens us to the natural flow of emotion, which is the flow of life itself.

QUESTIONS WATER AND YOU

These questions can help you feel the currents of Water in your life. Watch the movement of a river and imagine it flowing through your mind. Allow the answers to the questions to flow downstream with no hesitation.

1. How do you feel by the sea? By lakes? Rivers? Swamps?

2. How do you feel in winter?

3. Are you afraid of the dark?

4. Are you afraid of death?

5. What is your greatest fear?

6. Do you enjoy scary movies?

7. Do you seek danger?

8. How much salt do you want? How much salt do you eat?

9. Do you enjoy drinking water?

10. Are you a good swimmer?

11. What are your ambitions?

12. How do you feel when you have to do something you have never done before?

13. When has fear kept you from doing something you wanted to do?

14. When have you overcome your fears?

15. How do you feel in blue clothes? In a blue room?

16. When have you lost control of your bladder?

17. What or who inspires awe in you?

18. What makes you anxious?

19. What phobias have you had?

20. Do you fear the Divine?

21. When have you felt nervous?

22. When have you felt excited?

23. Do you enjoy roller coasters and other carnival rides?

24. What motivates you to get out of bed?

25. Do you meditate?

26. When have you trembled?

27. How do you feel in rainy weather?

28. Where does your tap water come from?

29. Where does your sewer water go?

30. How much water did you use today?

31. How much stress and anxiety is there in your life?

32. What feelings are you afraid of?

33. What situations make you nervous?

34. What do you do to relax and let go of stress?

35. When have you become emotionally numb?

36. When have you used alcohol, pharmaceuticals, or other drugs to help you cope with anxiety?

37. How much television do you watch? How much time do you spend per day on the computer?

38. Do you overwork?

39. How much thinking do you do?

As you consider the variety of responses to the questions, notice where your emotional responses to life flow freely and where they are constricted. Where do you feel most frightened? Close your eyes and feel yourself sink into the great river, the great energy flow of life. Allow it to take you into the depths of life's experience. After you've bathed in this source of your existence, give thanks to Water.

chapter 15

WOOD

Some say Dreamer's first dream was the elements. Out of His imagination sprang Fire, Earth, Metal, and Water, all surging in chaotic flux. After He finished His creation, Dreamer contemplated it and was pleased . . . for a while. Eventually, He got bored with the flux. Although it was pretty intriguing compared to sheer nothingness, flux didn't have much of a plot. In fact, with no here or there, no before or after, no you or me, one could say that flux has no plot at all. So it was that Dreamer began to long for some good stories to while away the eons. This is remarkable, considering stories hadn't been invented yet, and there was no one to tell them or act them out. But then Dreamer is remarkable.

One of Dreamer's many remarkable qualities is inventiveness, and He devised a way to generate a never-ending supply of really terrific tales: He dreamed a tree growing right at the center of his centerless universe.

Maybe you are thinking that a tree isn't much as a source of epic dramas, but things were different back then at the beginning. Once the tree was growing, it needed room to grow. Zap! Suddenly space existed where only chaos reigned before. And if this weren't enough, the tree needed its limbs to grow up and its roots to grow down. Zap again! Suddenly there was direction in the universe. Now that there was a way to get organized, the tree instructed Fire to put itself together as the sun above, and Earth got orders to collect itself as the soil below. Both Fire and Earth felt an agreeable sense of purpose once they were fitting into the new scheme of things, and it wasn't long before Metal and Water joined in, too.

Having created space and direction, the tree at the center of the universe began to grow. As it grew, it needed raw materials to make wood. It used what was at hand: Fire, Earth, Metal, and Water. These were organized into something new and unique: an individual self made of the elements, but somehow separate from them. This was the first protagonist.

As it continued to grow, the protagonist tree got older—that is, it moved into the future. Until now there had been no future to move into. With no growth and no development, nothing had ever happened, or at least nothing that would contrast with anything else. Each moment was indistinguishable from every other, and time was nonexistent. But the growth of the tree put an end to that. Now there was direction in time as well as in space, and the tree began to look ahead and plan how it would proceed with its growth. So the tree became the first visionary.

As the tree was growing and looking into the future, it foresaw the problem of death, and for that problem it came up with a fun solution: sex. Of course, sex requires the presence of another individual, so the tree asked Dreamer to dream up an appealing mate. In a trice, a second tree appeared nearby. The first tree became desperately infatuated and wanted to start reproducing immediately. The second tree had its own plans, though. It was more interested in branching out on its own personal growth before putting down roots and raising seedlings. Inevitably, the two quarreled, and the new tree stalked off. If it hadn't changed its mind, the universe would still be paralyzed with anger, but thankfully, the two got together and started a family.

So it was that Dreamer put a tree at the center of the universe, and from that tree were born time, space, individuality, conflict, sex, and death. It is no coincidence that these are the ingredients of a good yarn, and the first one the tree spun is still one of the best: boy meets girl, boy loses girl, boy gets girl back. Since then, every time a seedling sprouts, dozens of new stories sprout with it, so Dreamer hasn't been bored for a moment since.

It is springtime. A willow seed sprouts and starts growing up to be a tree. It will never be a blade of grass, never a trout or a termite. It will become a willow tree. It has the inner vision of willowness and will consult this vision like a blueprint at every occasion: "Hmm, let's see . . . We have good sunshine. Water supplies, minerals, and soil nutrients are holding up, so yes, there is an opportunity for further expansion. Shall we add some fins? Let's check the plan . . . No, no, not fins; we're supposed to be putting on wood. Willow wood at that."

Now the willow has to decide exactly how and where it will put the wood. Shall it grow low and bushy or tall and slender? Shall it grow straight, or shall it lean a bit this way or that to get more sunlight? Which of its branches shall grow first? Maybe they should all grow at the same time? There are thousands of decisions to be made.

I am not much different from a willow. I, too, am growing, consulting the vision I carry in my soul, and making decisions about how to make that vision into reality. There is this difference between the way willow grows and the way I do: willow's body keeps getting taller until her last day, whereas I achieved my full height many years ago. Whatever growth I have achieved since then has been in my mind and spirit. I have had a lot of growing to do in these areas, because my education stunted me.

My experiences in school were not exceptionally traumatic; in fact, I was a "successful" student. I say my education stunted me not because of what I had, but because of what I didn't have: initiation, a ritual that shows a person his or her purpose in life. In traditional societies this ritual is usually performed soon after puberty, because puberty marks the moment when physical growth is complete and education of the soul can begin. The perception of life purpose is the dawn of spiritual vision. There are many ways of performing the ritual, but it is always done under the guidance of elders. Often initiates are isolated from their families and undergo fasting and other hardships in the wilderness. Eventually they are visited by spirits who show them their life path and grant spiritual powers to help them along. The initiates return to society knowing how to contribute to their people. They are now young adults growing up to be elders themselves.[6]

Although I went through the outer form of initiation when I had my bar mitzvah, as a young man I was utterly ignorant. It didn't matter that I had a lot of formal education; without vision, I knew nothing I needed to know.

When I was in my twenties, my father often asked me when I was going to stop floundering. It made me furious to hear him say that. I maintained that I wasn't floundering, but he was right—I *was* floundering. Part of my fury was having to admit it. The other part was natural anger. I was not a young child anymore. I needed to find my direction in life, and no one was helping me.

Young children are not really concerned with their direction in life. The exciting question for them is, "What will I get for Christmas?" People getting close to initiation age sense life calling them to a bigger role. The exciting question then becomes, "What can I give for Christmas?" As they continue to grow, they realize Christmas goes on all year long and will keep going on after they die. The exciting question for the elder is "What can I give to Christmases seven generations from now?"

As discussed in chapter 11, anger arises to restore violated boundaries. When someone steps on your toe, for example, the emotion rises up and prompts you to restore the boundary. If your relationship to anger is good, a mild expression will do the trick: "Excuse me, but you are stepping on my toe." If you don't say anything at all or if your reaction is hostile or aggressive, your anger has been dammed up and has become out of balance.

Young people's spiritual boundaries need to grow; if they are denied the help they need, this is a boundary violation. Anger will naturally arise. If the young are seriously thwarted, anger can turn to violence. This happens in the ghettos, and these days in middle-class areas as well.

My own initiatory process was late, slow, and informal—a series of vision quests and other experiences over more than a decade, starting after I turned thirty. I was fortunate; many people today never find out what their purpose in life is. They have no way to express their gifts, and so each day is as monotonous and frustrating as the last.

Modern life opens a path not to the soul but to the shopping mall, and the force of growth has been diverted onto this path. The result is the growth of what we call the "gross national product," and unless it gets grosser every year, our "economy" founders. There is a word for out-of-control rapid growth: *cancer.* Cancer continues to spread in our bodies and on the earth because, like trees, we must have growth. The only way out is to rediscover that material growth is a youthful phase that prepares the way for real growth into elderhood.

In the short run, the prospects for rediscovery do not look good. The mass media show that we worship youth and want to prolong it as long as possible. The cruelty of this cult cuts deeper than the plastic surgeon's knife. Our culture throws elders on the scrap heap as soon as their prime consumer years are over.

I am not the only person angry about being kept in the dark. Deep down, most people resent the assumption that they were born to shop. This resentment is healthy, for anger provides power to overcome obstacles. It could destroy the whole frustrating economic system. An explosive change of this type is unlikely, though, because our frustration is enfeebled by denial and alcohol.

When George Bush, Sr., visited Russia as president of the United States, newspapers in this country carried front-page photos of him hoisting glasses of vodka with President Mikhail Gorbachev. Would it be conceivable that the two heads of state could publicly toast each other with a dangerous drug other than alcohol? Cocaine maybe, or heroin?

When the Spaniards arrived in Mexico five hundred years ago, they encountered a civilization much more advanced than their own. This civilization prized *pulque,* or agave wine, but drunkenness was severely punishable by law for anyone but the elderly. After destroying this civilization and subjecting its people to slavery, the Europeans introduced a long list of restrictive new laws. However, the invaders made distilled spirits available for the first time and removed any legal sanction against intoxication.

In order to understand the privileged place of alcohol in our society, we must note that the liver is the seat of the Wood element. The liver harbors the spiritual soul and is the source of vision, growth, and creativity. It is also the seat of anger. The plan for our life is to be found here. Alcohol devastates the liver. Years before cirrhosis sets in, the vision of the soul is lost. The alcoholic forgets what he or she is angry about. This may partially explain the epidemic of alcoholism among Native Americans. People who have been raped, beaten, robbed, massacred, and abused in every conceivable way are now taking out their rage on their own bodies and those of their spouses and children. But angry drunks are no problem compared to sober people who might remember the reasons for their anger. Thanks to alcohol, business goes on as usual at the mall.

Whatever your cultural heritage, if no one showed you your life's purpose, your spiritual development was neglected. It doesn't matter where your ancestors were born; the economic juggernaut packs the booze wherever it goes. You live in a nation of alcoholics. And business goes on as usual at the mall.

However snarled and hopeless the human dream gets, though, wild plants still willingly take people into their paradise. I don't know how they do that. It is a mystery I love to ponder and probably will never solve, which is fine with me because I like mysteries. I just keep asking the plants for their magic and admiring it when it comes.

Edna's life was snarled and hopeless when one of my colleagues brought her to see me. She said she had chronic fatigue syndrome; she had done very little but lie in bed for two years. The feeling she had was as if a giant were pinning her on the ground, making it impossible to move. This was her way of saying her Wood was thwarted and unable to grow, and the green tinge on her face, the shouting tone of her voice, her angry demeanor, and the rancid odor of her body confirmed this evaluation. After sharing my findings with Donna Guillemin, my colleague and former student, I left Edna in her care.

When I saw Edna again six months later, she was all smiles. "I've got some wild stories to tell you, Eliot," she said.

"Tell me," I said.

"Well, for one thing, you know I used to be violently allergic," Edna began.

"No, I don't think you told me that," I interrupted.

"Well, yes, I was. But after a few sessions with Donna, I noticed an amazing improvement. I said, 'Donna, what have you been giving me, anyway?' and she said that it was Scotch broom. 'Scotch broom?' I said, 'That stuff used to be my nemesis.' A while back I went into a restaurant and got a horrible asthma attack. I looked around, but I couldn't see anything that would set it off. So I asked the waiter if there was any Scotch broom around. He pointed way over to the other side of this huge room. There on the mantle was a tiny dried sprig of it. The waiter said it had been there for years. I couldn't breathe well enough to eat my meal, so I left, and the asthma went away almost immediately. When I told this story to Donna, I mentioned that since she started treating me, broom and I have become friends! And I went and stuck my face right into a big Scotch broom bush in full flower just to prove it! No ill effects whatsoever!

"Here's another thing," Edna continued, sticking her outstretched fingers in front of my face. Her fingernails were long, strong, and healthy-looking. Previously they had been yellow, rotting and disfigured with fungus growth. This was a significant sign, for according to Chinese physiology the health of the nails depends on the health of the liver.

"That's fantastic, Edna," I said, "but what about your fatigue?"

"Oh, that," she said. "No, I haven't been tired any more. In fact, for the first time I feel like I know what I'm supposed to be doing with my life, and I've gone back to school to start preparing for a new career."

QUESTIONS WOOD AND YOU

These questions can help you see how you grow. Stand with your back against a tall tree. Imagine that your spine is the trunk and your head is above the treetops. From this vantage point you can see the landscape of your whole life. Answer the questions clearly and truthfully.

1. How do you feel in spring?

2. What are your pet peeves?

3. When has it been difficult for you to make a decision?

4. How do you feel when your plans are thwarted?

5. When was the last time you shouted at someone?

6. When was the last time you wanted to shout at someone?

7. How do you feel in green clothes? In a green room?

8. Do you have a green thumb?

9. Is your closet organized? Your pockets? Purse? Desk?

10. Do you enjoy organizing people and events?

11. How coordinated are you?

12. How is your vision?

13. How are your fingernails and toenails?

14. How often do you drink alcohol? Why?

15. What frustrates you?

16. How do you feel in windy weather?

17. Do you enjoy sour, acid foods?

18. Have you ever been angry enough to cry?

19. How is your sense of direction?
    How are you at giving directions?

20. Did you have any developmental problems as a child?

21. What were the circumstances of your birth?

22. What are your experiences and feelings about childbirth?

23. How would you like your life to be five years from now?
    Ten years from now?

24. Do you have plans for your old age?

25. What creative activities do you enjoy? How often?

26. What new ideas or concepts have you come up with?

27. How are you a better person today than ten years ago?

28. What are your dreams in life? Your hopes for the future?

29. When have you felt full of hope?

30. How do you express frustration, irritation, and annoyance?

31. What are your personal boundaries?

32. What do you do when others are "out of bounds?"

33. When do you avoid expressing anger?

34. When has excessive anger moved you to aggression?

35. When has excessive anger made you hate someone?

36. In what circumstances have you been impatient?

37. When has clearly stating your boundaries kept you out of trouble?

30. What is the purpose of your life?

As you answer the questions, notice how responsive you are to the process of growth in your life at this moment. Like trees, we grow in different seasons and in different soils. What season of growth are you in right now? How fast or slow is it? What type of growth is it? What are the obstacles to your growth? How is the cycle of growth you are in now similar to that of some other period in your life?

Refocus on the tree you've been with. Ask this great teacher what you need to do to open your life more to growth and change within you. Visualize roots going down into the earth from your body next to this tree and then mentally draw leaves sprouting and blossoms and fruits coming forth from you. Rejoice that you are growing. Feel the frustration of the places in you where you are being thwarted. Touch the upward thrust of your life: Wood.

chapter 16

OTHER IMBALANCES

I n my approach to plant spirit medicine, most health concerns are understood as messengers of imbalanced relationship with the elemental forces of Fire, Earth, Metal, Water, or Wood. There are non-elemental imbalances as well, and here we will consider two of them: possession and the imbalance between masculine and feminine forces.

POSSESSION

The movies present sensationalized images of possession and exorcism, and this has caused many people to dismiss the phenomenon as nothing more than superstition. Possession is a real condition, though. The only form of medicine I have come across that does not recognize it is conventional Western medicine.

To understand possession, you can visualize the human body-mind-spirit as a complex of many vibrating parts that together produce a resonant field. Certain influences from outside, such as food, are brought in to enhance the resonance. Other influences are kept out because if allowed in they would damage the field or even destroy it. Our skin does a good job of excluding what is harmful. If you poured a vial of the human immunodeficiency virus (HIV) on your arm, it would not affect you at all as long as your skin was intact.

We also have what might be called an energetic skin, which keeps out dissonant mental and spiritual influences. Under exceptional duress, the energetic skin can sometimes be pierced by trauma or eroded by low-level stress. In either case, a harmful outside influence can enter. Like a guitar with one string out of tune or a computer with a virus, even a small dissonance can change the functioning of the whole. This is possession.

As life conditions have become more traumatic and stressful, I have seen more and more possessed people. Most of them would not make good stories for the sensationalist media because they usually lead what passes for normal lives.

The possessed person is not himself, so it is impossible to get through to him until the possession is removed. Occasionally people will identify the condition themselves. One young man, for example, said, "At times I hear a persuasive voice trying to convince me to do strange or destructive things." A young woman told me, "I don't believe in possession and all that nonsense, but if I did, I would say I am possessed. Ever since that car accident, I've been prone to depressions that just aren't like me." When these possessions were removed, the voices and depressive episodes disappeared.

For the most part, though, people are quite unaware of being possessed. They are usually also unaware that they cannot make rapport with others as they used to do, but that quality of being unnaturally shut off is the key to identifying the condition. Oftentimes the case history will point to a particular trauma or emotional stress that weakened the energetic "skin" and allowed the possession to enter.

What is the nature of the possessing influence? Is it a spirit entity? An emotional energy of some kind? A physical or spiritual toxin? In plant spirit medicine, we are not concerned with answering such questions. Our solution is to call upon plants to summon beneficial spirits that consume the invasive influence, whatever it may be. In Chinese medicine, the devouring beneficial spirits are called *dragons* because in that culture, dragons are creatures that bestow blessings. Their nature, too, remains a mystery, although their effectiveness cannot be denied.

HUSBAND-WIFE IMBALANCE

Another condition unknown to modern medicine is husband-wife imbalance. In a way, this is more serious than possession, because if unaddressed, it can cause premature death. To understand husband-wife imbalance, we can start by coming to terms with husband-wife *balance*. Everyone needs both masculine and feminine qualities to survive in this world. We need a bit of the active, aggressive go-getter, and we also need some of the nurturing, supportive, let-it-be attitude. These two should support each other, like the husband and wife in a marriage during ancient times. The husband has the muscle and temperament for the hunt. The wife is endowed by nature to care for the family: she has the breasts and temperament to feed the young.

As long as husband and wife are true to their respective natures, the family thrives. This is husband and wife in balance with each other. But imagine what would happen if one day the husband comes home, flops himself down on a hide, and says to his wife, "Honey, I'm sick and tired of chasing mammoths. No sooner do I drag one home than you guys devour it and I have to go out and find another one. I've had it! From now on I'm going to stay around the fire and take it easy, like you. You go out and bring home the meat!" The wife might do quite well out hunting with the boys, but what would happen to the young ones at home? With no breast to turn to, they would soon starve to death. If this went on long enough, the family would die of a husband-wife imbalance. And if the wife suddenly announced she was sick of being oppressed, sick of staying around the camp, and from now on she was darn well going to insist on her right to have fun killing animals like her husband, the result would be the same: death by husband-wife imbalance.

Before I make myself persona non grata with the women's movement and the men's movement alike, remember this: I insist that everyone, whether man or woman, has both husband and wife characteristics. We all have to be part hunter, part nurturer.

Often a person who is suffering from husband-wife imbalance will sense that death is near—long before there is any medical reason to think so. As the masculine, aggressive principle weakens and resigns itself, the person loses vitality. Glenda, a sixty-year-old housewife, came to me in this condition. Her fatigue was so great she could barely move. Medical doctors had found that an antibody was destroying her thyroid hormone as fast as it could be formed, but they were unable to correct the problem. A host of nonconventional therapists had no success either. As she climbed onto my treatment couch, Glenda confessed in a whisper that she felt she was not long for this world. From my perspective, her thyroid hormone was a carrier of the "husband" principle that provided the get-up-and-go to restart her life and work. As soon as my plant friends got husband and wife to stop fighting over the thyroid secretions, she was full of vitality again.

Bob, another client of mine, was an airline pilot who complained, "Nothing seems to matter to me anymore. Life doesn't interest me. When I'm not working, I just lie around all the time. This isn't like me. I've always been a happy, highly motivated kind of guy. I enjoyed work, and I enjoyed working on projects at home when I wasn't flying.

"I have some physical complaints, too," Bob continued. "I'm eating huge amounts of food. I'm hungry all the time, but I just don't seem to get the value out of what I'm eating. Also, my wife and I have been trying to have a baby, but no luck. The doctors checked us both out. She's okay, but my sperm count is just about nonexistent. This worries me a lot, and yet sometimes I think maybe it's for the best that we haven't had a baby, because ever since I haven't been feeling well, I can't tolerate my wife. She can say just the simplest little thing, and it throws me into a blind rage. I can't control myself."

Bob's symptoms dramatized the state of the broken inner marriage. The husband within was henpecked, impotent, and enraged at his inner wife, who was letting her husband go hungry. Correcting the inner husband-wife imbalance had dramatic results. Bob came back five days after the treatment, and I recorded his words verbatim:

The change in me is indescribable! The moment I walked out of here last time, I burst into laughter! I couldn't stop laughing! What a relief! I've finally come back to life. I've got my energy back, and I've been working around the house again. I haven't noticed the hunger so much, and I haven't lost my temper with my wife.

Within six weeks, Bob had his sperm count taken again. It was more than four times what it was before the plant spirits brought his husband and wife together again.

chapter 17

~~~~~~~~

REMEDIES

Gil Milner was a distinguished physician with an impressive list of credentials. Among other things, he was a neurologist, a psychiatrist, a child psychiatrist, and a professor of medicine at a major university. Years ago he attended one of my trainings. I couldn't help but wonder how a person with his background would relate to the spirits of plants, so after each dream journey I peeked over his shoulder to see what he was writing in his notebook. In each case, I saw esoteric-looking squiggles with syllables jotted below them in a foreign language.

After several days, my curiosity overcame my embarrassment about peeking. "What is that strange stuff you write in your notebook, Gil?" I asked.

"Oh, you know, it's the song of the plant," he answered.

"How's that?"

"Well, each plant gives you its power in the form of a song, right?"

"I don't know. Does it?" I asked.

"Sure! Don't they sing to you?"

"No. They haven't yet."

"Hmm, I thought they did that with everybody. Look, this is a kind of notation to remember the melody, and these are the words of the song written underneath," said Dr. Milner, showing me his notebook.

On the final day of the course, after the students had treated each other, I approached him. "Everyone has been treated now except me," I said. "I would like to ask you for a treatment."

"Yes, of course. I would be happy to treat you," he replied.

I said, "I want you to sing me my medicine."

The doctor blushed, looked at his feet, and stammered something incoherent. Looking up again, he saw I was determined. He nodded, and I lay down on the treatment table so he could interview me and take my pulses. After that procedure, he disappeared into the next room with the other students to discuss what plant should be sung. A few minutes later they reappeared. He picked up my drum and played a slow, loping rhythm and then began to sing a repetitive, strangely beautiful chant. It was absolutely authoritative. I felt the song enter my chest. Tears came to my eyes. Dr. Milner picked up the tempo and lifted my mood; I smiled. He stopped singing and checked my pulses, and then all the students once again went into the next room to consult.

When they returned, he drummed and chanted as before, but this time the effect was deeper, more internal. I closed my eyes and suddenly lost consciousness of everything in the room. I found myself in the woods, sitting on a forest floor that was carpeted with wild ginger. The song of the ginger was pouring out of the mouths of its purple flowers, offering me treasures: heart-shaped leaves, rich soil, breezes sighing in the graceful arms of maples, and certain other wordless blessings.

Gil stopped singing, and I returned to the classroom. "Wild ginger," I said. "Asarum canadense." He nodded and checked my pulse, even though he must have already known that a splendid treatment had been done. I got up and gave him a hug to express my thanks. His face was red, his eyes full of tears, and he trembled noticeably.

"How are you doing?" I asked.

"Wherever I travel," he said, "the shamans always seek me out. They give me their feathers. I've got a whole drawer full of them at home. I could never figure out why the shamans do that. 'I'm a doctor,' I would say to myself. 'I'm not going to use their kind of medicine.' But now I know why."

Plant spirit medicine is a magico-religious rite in which plant gods bestow their grace. How is that grace invoked? Some people use song; others use pills and potions; still others lay on hands, wave feathers, or dance. Who knows how many ways may be waiting to be discovered or rediscovered?

Whatever method is used, the spirits are invited to help the patient enter the dream of nature; this has nothing to do with fighting illness. For us, there is no such thing as an herb that is good for arthritis or migraine or depression or cancer. Whatever medicine a plant spirit gives you, that's what it will do for your patients. As the Matsés Indians in the Amazon told Peter Gorman, if you want to use a plant for healing, you have to dream it, or it won't work for you. Rarely do two people have exactly the same dreams. Rarely do two people use the same plant in exactly the same way.

Even conventional herbalists will privately admit that their art is highly personal. The successes of one herbalist cannot be duplicated by another using the same remedies. Homeopathic herbalism is an exception.

Homeopathy is a healing method that employs rigorous empirical methods to discover which symptoms a given medicine will provoke. Samuel Hahnemann, the founder of homeopathy, considered plants to be "morbific agents" given to bring on an artificial disease similar to the natural one the patient suffers from. This stimulates the patient's recuperative powers, helping them to overcome both diseases very quickly. While homeopathy is highly effective when skillfully applied, it relates to plants and healing in a different way than that of plant spirit medicine.

The Bach Flower Remedies are an outgrowth of homeopathy. Edward Bach, an English homeopathic physician, was sensitive to the power of plants to heal what he called "negative" emotional states. He set out to create a simple system of medicine that could be practiced by anyone without special training, and he succeeded. By contrast, plant spirit medicine students must go through years of specialized training before they are prepared to deliver all the medicine has to offer.

I find that self-healing with plants is rarely effective. Self-healing does sometimes occur, but it is the exception rather than the rule, because illness takes root in our emotional blind spot. Disease is a call for help, and often the best way to help ourself is to accept the help of others. Exaggerated independence is one of the attitudes that isolates us and makes us ill. Healing can be a celebration of our connectedness and interdependence.

Michael Harner tells an anecdote about an Indian shaman he met in the Amazon during the 1950s. Harner was impressed by the young man's power, and he also enjoyed his company. The two became friends. Before

Michael's return to the United States, he invited his friend to make shamanic dream journeys to Berkeley so they could continue their friendship. Much to Michael's surprise, the powerful shaman appeared crestfallen.

"I cannot do this," he said.

"Why not?" Michael asked. "I've seen you do much greater things!"

The Indian replied, "I cannot visit you in Berkeley because I do not know the trails." This was his way of saying there is no substitute for experience.

The same thing holds true for someone who wants to learn the medicine of plants: there is no substitute for experience. This medicine comes from intimacy with living plants. Just as no one would think of trying to make babies with a character in a novel, no one should think of trying to make medicine with a plant in a book—not even this book. I will describe some of my intimacies, but yours would be different.

One of my favorite plants for helping with Fire imbalance is scarlet pimpernel, *Anagallis arvensis*. This is a familiar wayside plant in America, Europe, and other parts of the world. It is a low, sprawling herb with tiny flowers that are usually salmon-colored with a magenta center and bright-yellow stamens. They open in sunny weather and close tight when it is dark or cloudy. The taste of this herb is bitter and offensive and is said to be somewhat poisonous. All in all, this is a difficult plant to get intimate with, but well worth the effort. In English herbalism, it had a reputation for dispelling melancholy, and Somerset folk still know it as "Laughter Bringer."

My dream journey to the spirit of this plant took me through long stretches of cold, dark space until I arrived at a small, distant planet. The sphere seemed deserted until I got to the remotest part, where I saw a gruff, unshaven man dressed in a tight T-shirt and black pants.

"Are you the spirit of scarlet pimpernel?" I asked.

"What's it to ya?"

"Well, I . . ."

"Listen, buddy, why don't you just take off to the next solar system. There's some nice flowers over there. Scram."

This had to be the spirit of scarlet pimpernel! He was showing the same bitterness and the same over-protectiveness in the dream as he did in waking reality. I remembered that the warmth of the sun would get him to open up and share his beauty.

"I love your flowers!" I said. "They have the wildest color combination! It makes me happy to look at them! You must be a beautiful guy behind that gruff front!" He cracked a little smile and blushed. I went on, "What are you doing here all alone on this frigid little planet?"

A tear trickled down the tough guy's cheek. "People are so cold, so heartless!" he said. "They can hurt you if you let your guard down. I take everything to heart—I'm just too vulnerable, I guess."

He didn't need to say more to let me know he had medicine for the heart protector. When he saw I understood his act, he threw back his head and laughed uninhibitedly.

"May I use you?" I asked. "Will you share your medicine with others?"

In reply he took my hands, and we danced in a circle, abandoning ourselves to joy.

Mullein, *Verbascum thapsus,* is another herb common in both the New World and the Old. The leaves are soft, fuzzy, and flannel-like. Second-year plants put up a tall central stalk tipped with bright-yellow, sweet-smelling flowers. A warm infusion of these flowers in olive oil is used as eardrops for children's earaches.

Often in my dreams of plants, I see nothing and hear nothing, yet I experience a definite inner sensation. If the sensation is disagreeable, I assume the plant can heal it; if it is agreeable, I assume the plant spirit is showing me the benefits it has to offer. My dream with mullein was this way. Nothing seemed to happen, yet I felt coddled and secure, as if my mother had just given me warm milk, tucked me into bed with mullein-flannel sheets, and sung me a sweet lullaby. Since that time, I have used mullein to bring comfort and security to many people who suffered from imbalance of Earth.

Plantain (*Plantago* ssp.) is a native of Europe that has accompanied the European peoples in the colonization of the world. Some Native American tribes referred to this plant as "white man's footsteps," because it was found wherever the newcomers trod. It is a soft, bland plant whose young leaves can be eaten as salad. This softness is balanced by tremendous strength; plantain competes well among the toughest grasses. In fact, if you live in a temperate climate, you probably have plantain growing in your lawn or the nearest park.

Plantago psyllium is the source of psyllium seeds, which constitute the main ingredient in many commercial bulk laxatives. Plantain has many other uses among folk herbalists. It has been a favorite of mine since my

147

farm days in Vermont because the juice, when introduced into a suppurating lesion, will eliminate most of the infection and inflammation within twenty-four hours.

As I already mentioned, plantain was the first plant I dreamed with. The spirit appeared to me as a winged fairy holding a magic wand in one hand and a vial of sleeping potion in the other. I could use her medicine, she said, for the mental and spiritual equivalents of pus and constipation. She called herself a gentle but powerful purifier of the soul. She let me know she could bring purity and sparkle where old filth had polluted the mind; thus, her strongest affinity is to the Metal element and the colon in particular. When such problems cause insomnia, her medicine is doubly indicated.

The stream orchids of western North America and the helleborine orchids of eastern North America and Europe all belong to the genus *Epipactis* and all have similar medicine. Visiting the live plant, I enjoyed the complex beauty of the flowers, but I was even more struck with an unusual sensation I felt when grasping the leaf. It was as if the plant were holding my hand in a reassuring way. Here's what I wrote in my notebook after my dream with *Epipactis gigantea*:

> The stream orchid is a very companionable spirit, like an old and trusted friend. There is no need to speak with it, for we understand each other so well. Telepathically it told me that this is an elixir for loneliness, fear, and agitation coming from imbalances of the Water element. Its effect is a deeply calming presence, like viewing a still pond in tranquility with my life's companion by my side. This spirit is completely loyal, a reliable aid for separation anxiety.
>
> Its action comes from its willingness to share the peace of its home. The plant is made of the vibrations that surround it. Observe well the home it selects: moist, shady, undisturbed. It only grows in magical places, feeding on peace and storing it in its flesh.

Throughout the world, pussy willow is the messenger of spring, foretelling the rebirth of nature. Willows (*Salix* ssp.) make medicine for the Wood element.

Indeed, these trees offer a wonderful example of the qualities of Wood in balance. Anyone who has worked with willow knows that it bends when other woods break. On the other hand, the sheer strength of the growth force in the willow is unsurpassed. A dry stick inserted into moist soil will sprout roots and leaves.

To those whose Wood has become rigid and who are frustrated, uptight, or clumsy, willow brings grace and flexibility. To the drifters, the hopeless, and the stunted whose Wood has become feeble, the willow spirit brings a surge of power, a vision of the future, and new growth.

Another category of plant spirit medicines is comprised of those that bring something special to the spirit without having any particular elemental correspondence. There is a varied range of effects available from these remedies. I will mention just some of my favorites.

Mugwort is highly regarded wherever it is found. It is indispensable to the acupuncturist's art. Small cones of dried mugwort are burned at acupuncture points on the body to stimulate the patient's vitality. Among some Native Americans of California, it is a sacred plant of divination and spiritual healing. It is important in Mesoamerican folk medicine. In certain European traditions, sprigs of the herb are placed under the pillow to provoke vivid dreams, and the plant has been linked with the practice of magic since Anglo-Saxon times.

In plant spirit medicine, mugwort also occupies a prominent position, for it is the most important of the remedies that are used to effect transfers of energy within the meridian system. These transfers are called for in many instances. For example, sometimes energy can get blocked as it flows from one meridian to the next. It can also happen that the energy in one side of the body becomes markedly less than the energy on the other side, causing lopsided functioning. Both problems can be detected through skillful reading of the Chinese pulses, and both are remedied by the mugwort spirit.

Here is a transcription of my initial field notes on wood anemone (*Anemone lyallii* in the West, *Anemone quinquefolia* in the East, and *Anemone nemorosa* in Europe):

A slender nymph or gnome appeared and flew silently away. I followed. We landed on a rock ledge and waited quietly for the right moment. It led me through a narrow cleft. Inside there was a cave, which opened into a large room with a stone idol in the center.

The idol came to life and got on its hands and knees, giving me a ride on its back. It turned into a turtle and walked serenely to the river. We plunged in and stayed on the bottom.

An enigmatic journey, but I think the point is this: The problems and cares of life loom like the cedars and firs of the forest where the lowly anemone lives. Entering the world of the plant spirits requires lightness, quickness, and timing so that you can slip unnoticed through the cracks of the rock or ordinary waking state. So anemone is to be used before another remedy, particularly when the patient is insensitive or preoccupied with worldly problems. This will lead the second remedy into the patient's cave (skull) and introduce it to the stone idol (god of his consciousness). Then the two can play together at the bottom of the stream (of awareness).

St. Johnswort (*Hypericum perforatum*) is a perennial favorite of herbalists and plant magicians. Every medical system throughout the ages has found a use for this herb. It was a vulnerary (used for treating wounds) for Christian forces during the Crusades. Currently, St. Johnswort is in vogue as an antidepressant in European herbalism; its earlier fame was as an exorcist. In homeopathy, hypericum is the *sine qua non* for nerve damage of all kinds. Only in the American West, where St. Johnswort is known as Klamath weed, is it not revered; on the contrary, this herb is the target of chemical eradication campaigns because it invades pasture and range land.

My dream of St. Johnswort was short and simple. A disembodied voice told me, "I will bind together that which has been rent asunder." Since that time, I have used it as cement for fractured souls. It works wonders in cases such as the following.

A woman in her early twenties consulted me with complaints of severe fatigue that had started several months before. Previously, she had been active and energetic. In questioning her, I discovered that in the nine months before the onset of her illness, the woman had two abortions. Her boyfriend was very supportive, she said, and they both agreed this was the best thing to do. She said she loved her boyfriend and they planned to have children later. Her voice sounded quite even as she reported that she had no issues with the abortions. But this was just her mind reporting.

Her spirit was saying that it was devastated by the loss of two children in such a short time, and it was presenting fatigue to prove it.

It was clear that this young woman would not get well while her mind and spirit were split apart, so I called on St. Johnswort to close the gap. The instant she received the St. Johnswort spirit, she sat bolt upright on the treatment table, her dull eyes suddenly gleaming. "Wow! I feel terrific!" she said.

Another plant helped me discover how to deliver the medicine of the spirits. In the beginning of my practice, I had homeopathic preparations made of each plant I used as medicine, and these preparations served as a carrier to deliver the healing spirits to my patients. Later on, I began to use the services of *Erodium cicutarium,* otherwise known as filaree or storksbill.

Filaree is a pretty little plant commonly found in disturbed soil in temperate areas around the world. It has lacy, fernlike leaves and magenta, star-shaped flowers. The spirit of this plant offered itself to me as a kind of spiritual messenger service. I couldn't imagine why I would need a messenger until the U.S. Food and Drug Administration cut off the supply of my homeopathic remedies. I returned to the filaree spirit and asked if it could summon the spirits of other plants I might need to help heal my patients. The spirit said it would be delighted to do this. It was hard for me to believe this would work, but I either had to take him at his word or abandon plant spirit medicine altogether. I accepted his offer and found filaree delivers a purer, more specific medicine than the laboratory does.

Since that time, I have experimented with various methods of preparing filaree to use in treatment: homeopathic potentization, radionics, flower essences, and others. I have asked my messenger to bring plant spirits through my hands into my patient's body. All these methods work well. For years now, I have exclusively used the hands-on method, asking my messenger to summon whatever plant spirit is needed at the time.

part three

MEDICINE DREAMS
OF THE HEALERS

chapter 18

DON ENRIQUE SALMÓN

I
n the process of writing this book, I confirmed something I had suspected since beginning my work with plants: I did not invent plant
spirit medicine. All around the world there are people who heal with
the spirits of plants. This is one of the great medical traditions of the planet.

Why had I never heard of plant spirit medicine before? Generations
of ethnobotanists had catalogued the practices of plant healers in every
corner of the earth, and yet before I wrote the first edition of this book,
there was no literature on their spiritual healing practices unless they
happened to use "psychoactive" plants. Is the spirit bound to only a few
psychoactive molecules? Will social scientists ever be able to admit that
every plant is a miracle and a mystery? In looking for ways to avoid ecological cataclysm, will modern humanity take the time to learn from our
plant brothers and sisters how to live successfully on the earth? If we do
so soon, we may find that there are still a few plant healers left who can
introduce us to vegetable wisdom.

In this section of the book, we will meet four such people. Each has
his or her own way of relating to the spirit power of plants, yet each story
elaborates on the same themes: dreams, pilgrimage, and vision quest as
reliable sources of knowledge; the willingness of plant spirits to teach and

heal humankind; the journey to the Underworld; the importance of individualized and nonroutine treatment of patients; the power and aliveness of the elements; and the importance of gratitude and humility.

Our first plant healer is Enrique Salmón, a young man of a Mexican tribe known as the Rarámuri, or Tarahumara. Don Enrique grew up in Southern California and was trained in the traditions of his people by his parents and grandparents. Fluent in English, Spanish, and Rarámuri, he is uniquely well equipped to interpret ancient wisdom to modern people.

The interview that follows took place near his home in the American Southwest.

Eliot: Tell me how you learned some of the things you know about plant spirits.

Enrique: Well, growing up it was my grandparents being around, and my mom always teaching me things about plants. As a little kid, the way I was brought up, we used plants instead of going to a doctor for healing. I was told by my grandparents when I was about twelve that they were going to teach me about plants. I did not really care about it at the time. I was busy with other things, just being a kid. But they started teaching me.

Eliot: So your training as a shaman started with plants?

Enrique: Yes. What plants are good for—what illnesses and that sort of thing. [My grandparents] waited for a while, until I got a little more mature, before they started to be concerned with how to get in touch with the spirits within the plants. They taught me certain songs and certain ways to pick the plants and to pray to the plants and the earth, to bring out more of the medicine in a plant.

Eliot: And that's what the songs were for?

Enrique: The songs are to the plants and to the earth also, to get the medicine out of the plant to help the patient more.

Asking the plant for its help. Asking for it to do what
it naturally does, for what it was put here for. As I got
older, I kept learning different things, and eventually
my grandfather started to teach me more about spiritual
healing—how to get in touch with the spirits that are
around us all the time and those spirits that get inside
of someone who is possessed by a spirit or from a witch
or a sorcerer. I learned about that. I learned about protecting those people and then healing those people with
the use of the spirits. Because the spirits are out there
just waiting to help us. We've got to use the right words
or the songs to get them to help out a little.

So I learned that for a while, until I was eighteen.
Then I moved away from home. By that time I was
fairly accomplished, but I still had a lot to learn.

I picked up some more when I was in New Mexico
on the Navajo land. They talked more about divination. It was a different technique to tell what is wrong
with a person. Then this Oglala Sioux guy taught me a
lot about the Four Directions and how to be in contact
with those spirits. Then frequent trips down into Chi-
huahua [Mexico] and learning some more by watching
and asking a lot of questions with healers down there.

So that is pretty much the extent of my education
that got me here so far. I am still learning. I still pick
up things. I am still asking a lot of questions.

Eliot: Is there anything you would like to say about specific
individual plants? How you used them to help other
people? What you have learned from them?

Enrique: My plant spirit helper is what we call *chuchupate,* or the
Mexicans call it *osha.* It is a very powerful plant, but
also a very forgiving plant. What I mean is, some plants
are very strong as medicine. [Osha] is very strong, but
it doesn't do anything to you on the side. I use it for
infections, cuts, arthritis, headaches, sore throats, colds,

stomachaches. It cures almost anything. You make a strong tea or just take the root and chew it. It tastes awful. I always carry a piece with me. It repels rattle-snakes and witches. You have to watch out for those witches. You never know when they are going to be around the next corner. Osha talks to me sometimes.

Eliot: Does it?

Enrique: Yes. The root. The whole plant will talk, but I get more messages from the root.

Eliot: What are the things it says to you?

Enrique: It helps me figure out what is wrong with people. If I have a problem with a patient and I'm not quite sure what to do, I can go to osha. It will tell me. It will help me figure out what plants it can work with. Also, osha will let me know when I am getting in too deep in a problem.

Eliot: Someone else's problem or your own?

Enrique: Someone else's problems do become my own, especially when I am working with spells, when people have become possessed by something. Osha will tell me, "Hey, take it easy here!" or it will help me figure out how to go about a ceremony.

There was one instance where a woman had a bad back. She went to doctors, and they could not do anything, so she came to me. Osha told me to do something I have never done before or since: to draw this particular design on the ground and have her sit on it. I can't even remember what this drawing was any more. I know it had a big circle with little half circles around it. So that's one way osha will help out. Some-times it will say, "You can't help this person. You are not strong enough yet." So it is my plant spirit helper.

Eliot: How do you go about putting yourself into the state of mind to receive those communications from plants?

Enrique: I try and find a quiet place to relax for a few hours. I can do it at home, but it's better outside. I'm not really thinking much about other things. I will drink some of the tea from the plant and get the plant itself. This is what is weird: I work with plants that have been picked. The spirits inside stay alive. I drink some of the tea, then I wait for something to happen. I'll do it right before I go to sleep, and wait for a dream. Or I will do it in the middle of the day and sit there and hum a little medicine song. I close my eyes, and the spirit will come to me. It really doesn't look like a person to me. Usually it's animals. The animal will come, and I hear the voice in Rarámuri say, "Hi, how are you doing? This is who I am. Do you have any questions?" I will ask the question, and they will answer. Sometimes they say, "Oh, I can't tell you that right now," or "You are not ready for that right now," or "Maybe when you are fifty years old. Right now you are too young," or something like that. They are generally good messages that help me to figure out how to use a plant. Sometimes they don't tell me much of anything. But it's always a very positive experience.

Eliot: Is that a method you developed yourself, or did your grandfather show you how to do it?

Enrique: My grandmother showed me her way of doing it, which is different. She would talk to the live plants, touch them, and just sit there. I developed this other way because I was in the service, then I was in college. I didn't always have the time to go out into the countryside to meet the plants. That's where I found the spirits are still in the plants after you picked them and they dried up. Not for very long though. Maybe after eight months they are not there any more. So I incorporated the chanting. That is something I learned from my grandfather; he always used to sing. So I incorporated what I learned from both my grandparents. It's just something that works for me—very powerful.

Eliot: When you are using the healing power of plant spirits, do you always have your patient eat or drink some part of the plant?

Enrique: Sometimes the spirits will tell me to combine certain plants to use as a smoking ritual.

Eliot: For you to smoke?

Enrique: Yes, for me to smoke and blow onto the patient. The spirit of the plant comes out in a visible form and goes into the patient to make them stronger.

Eliot: Have you done healing at a distance with plant spirits?

Enrique: Using corn, I have done healing at a distance. There was a friend of mine—can't remember what tribe he was from—who was going to court one day, and he asked me the night before if I would do something to make the situation at court a positive one for everyone. He told me the time they were going to meet at this court place, and at the same time I went outside, using corn meal and a couple of songs. Corn is a very positive plant—healing all sorts of ways—so I used the corn to make things good there. It worked. Everybody came out winning. He said when it was all over, they came out still friends. To this day, things still work out.

Eliot: What about songs? Have the plants taught you any songs?

Enrique: Yes. The plants have taught me a few songs. I forgot a couple of them. They were songs I used for a particular instance. There is one general song that I was taught that I use all the time in working with plants.

Eliot: It was taught by . . . ?

Enrique: By my grandfather. It is a very simple song. Tarahumara songs are redundant. The people in the ceremony get restless because I keep on repeating it. When I sing the song right now, it's not going to do anything; it has to be in a different situation. "Hey hey hey hey"—that's it. It's just the spirit of the song that I learned from my grandfather. It's a general cure-all song.

There are some more specific songs for other occasions. Like when I'm healing a place or a whole family—that song is like, "Hey ya ho ya hey ya ho." It keeps on repeating like that.

[Lifts up his pant legs and inspects his shins.] I've got a lot of bugs on my legs. It must be the cream I put on.

Eliot: *[Waving off insects.]* I've got a few of them, too.

Enrique: They are always after me. I must have good medicine or something. I'm trying to remember a plant song. Listen to this—it is not a typical Tarahumara song at all: "Hey hey hey hey." That one was in conjunction with sagebrush. The sage was telling me to sing this song. I was using it for a spiritual cleansing on a friend of mine. He had a hard time. For a while there, he had these witches after him. I used that song a lot. I haven't used it since he left. I guess it was just a song for him.

Eliot: Is there anything else you want to talk about?

Enrique: For a long time, I would only work with Native Americans and Hispanics because I thought they understood where I was coming from, that would make it work. If someone comes in off the street who has always gone to white-man doctors and they want me to heal them using spirit medicine, it probably is not going to work—or that's what I thought for a long time.

But then I had a vision. I was on a medicine quest three years ago, on the side of this mountain range by myself, seeking some more medicine, some more ideas, singing songs and smoking things—nothing hallucinogenic, just smoking certain plants and waiting for something to happen. A bear was hanging around a lot, but he was just there to protect me from what might harm me because I was there by myself. I was getting a lot of messages from the deer. Finally it came to me in a dream from the deer that I was not going to get any new medicine from this quest. "What I'm going to give you is a path to follow. Not a new path, but something to add on to the path you are on already." It was to pass on some approaches to the spirit world for white people.

Native Americans have their way of finding out things. If a big storm comes along, Native Americans' roots are deep into the earth. We are still going to be here. But for a lot of Anglos, there aren't many roots. The next storm comes along, and they would all be blown off the universe.

I was told to help out these people any way I can—how to approach the spirit world, how a Native American develops roots into the earth. The only way I can think about how to do it is what we are doing right now. Tell people how to go about learning things, how I get messages from the plants, from the spirits. Maybe someone can read your book and learn a few more things, a few more ideas. Because the traditions are missing.

My way isn't going to work for everybody. The Tarahumara ways aren't going to work for white people or Apaches or whatever because there is this mind-set that comes with traditions. I think that the best way for Anglos is not to adopt our traditional ways, but to learn from us how traditions work. Then put these together and say, "Okay, how does this work? How can this work for us?"

Eliot: I guess that's basically what I'm doing.

Enrique: Yeah! Yeah! That's why I like what you are up to.

Eliot: A typical white person, if he wants to learn something about plants, will go to a university and read a lot of books and listen to lectures of other people who have read books.

Enrique: That is a different way of knowing.

Eliot: That's right! I would like you to talk a little bit about your way of knowing.

Enrique: I am sort of an enigma myself.

Eliot: I mean the knowing of your people.

Enrique: Okay. To a Tarahumara, knowing something has nothing to do with being able to use the scientific name of the plant. Americans like to put everything in their own little boxes. For the Tarahumara or Rarámuri, everything interconnects; you can't really put something into its own little box. That would be to kill it, to cut it off. It has these big root systems throughout the universe. To take one part of this root system and put it in a box to classify it is to kill it. Everything is interconnected.

Eliot: How does a Tarahumara go about learning about plants?

Enrique: We Tarahumaras have our basic education as we are growing up. It has nothing to do with reading books. We learn how to use particular plants for healing, for food, for drinks. We're taught by example—taught about how to farm particular plants.

Now, if a Tarahumara wants to learn a little bit more than the average person, he has to get in contact with the spirits and wait for a dream. That dream takes him into the real world. We don't live in the real world here. This is a flesh-and-blood world, not the real world. The real world is where the spirit of osha comes and talks to me. The real world isn't in the technology or all those books. It's in our visions and dreams. Whenever we dream or have a vision, a door is opening for us. If we learn something from that, that's when we actually know something. That is "knowing." That's how it works.

If I want to know more than the normal Tarahumara knows, I have to experience that through visions and dreams. Not every Tarahumara does that. We are born with different paths. Some of us were made to be good farmers. Some of us are put here to be healers. Some are put here to be good basket-makers.

Some Tarahumaras have become Christians or Catholics. Those that become Catholics, that is no big deal. Catholicism is really cool because it does sort of ritualize. That ritual takes you to this other realm, and so that's good. Jehovah's Witnesses and Protestants take the Tarahumara away from the real knowing, because knowing to the Christians is this book—the Bible. But knowing is not in the written words, not in the book. That is what scientists do. Traditional Tarahumaras still respect this other way of knowing things. Some Tarahumaras will travel days to go to a person they respect to have that person help them out to learn things.

Eliot: Are these "knowers" the most respected people among the Tarahumara?

Enrique: Yes! They are the older people who have been around for a while [and] who have taken the time to learn these things and to pass this information on and keep traditions around. I was thinking about my mom, for example. She didn't finish school, but she is one of the wisest people I know. If someone from the university were to categorize her, she would be at the bottom of the list. But that is in white man's society. If I were to take her to [the] Hopi, for example, where they still respect the old ways, she would be considered a very intelligent person, very wise, because she knows a lot in that tradition. They would look at her and say, "Gosh, she can cook traditional foods. Take them right out of the earth. She doesn't need to go to Safeway. She can make these baskets. She knows about all these medicines." What more could you ask for? That's great! That is a lifetime of learning!

Most Americans don't understand that other sense of knowledge. Knowledge to Americans is being able to recite Shakespeare from memory, to split up an atom, or something like that. But what does that do for you except being able to write papers to impress these other people who don't know what they're talking about either? I'm getting my PhD, but those three little letters are not going to make me a stronger healer. They are not going to help me learn more about herbs or be able to pick corn off the stalk and make it into tortillas. All it's going to do is when I write articles or a book, people are going to be willing to read it. It is kind of sad.

Eliot: I wanted to ask you about something entirely different. Do you have anything to say about using local plants versus using plants that grow somewhere else?

Enrique: When I'm healing someone, I prefer to use plants from the area where the person lives. A person living in this area is in contact with these plants around them. These plants are affecting them, and they don't realize it. These plants are tough. They send out these messages. A lot of the people that have been here for a long time, they seem like the plants out here. They are tough people. They realize it's a tough environment, but they endure it because they love it. It becomes a part of them. So that's why I like to use plants from a person's environment as much as I can. Even have the person pick the plants that I'm going to use in the ceremony. I think it helps them feel the medicine spirit of the plant to know where the medicine is coming from. A lot of white-man medicines, you don't know where it comes from. It comes from some lab. Sometimes they do come from the plants, but they have pretty much killed the spirit of the plant by the time they turn it into a pill or some liquid in a jar. The chemicals are there, I guess, but they are not live chemicals. In that sense, I try to use most plants from their environment.

chapter 19

DON LUCIO CAMPOS

t was the Nahua Indian herbalist doña Modesta Lavana Pérez who told me where don Lucio Campos lived. My friend John had been seeking help for some health concerns, so I took him to doña Modesta's house in Morelos, Mexico. John lay on a mat in the sun while she prayed over him and rubbed fresh herbs into his skin. When the healing was over, my friend rested quietly while doña Modesta and I chatted.

"People from your country come here wanting me to teach them about herbs," she said, "but they are always looking for herbs to treat certain diseases. They say, 'And this disease, doña Modesta, what plant is there for this disease?' I tell them, 'There are no herbs for specific illnesses.' Then they say, 'There has to be a plant for this problem.' So I tell them, 'Well, if there has to be a plant for this problem, then go out and find it yourself!'"

She laughed, and continued, "I use the same plants for everything: the same ones my mother used. When she was alive, she was the best healer in the village; now I am the best."

"Doña Modesta," I asked her, "how much of the healing is performed by the spirit of the plants?"

"A lot. The juice of the plants is their blood. The blood captures the healing power of the sun. When I pick them, our brothers the plants sacrifice themselves to share that power with us."

"Doña, I am learning a little bit about plant medicine myself, but my mother did not teach me, as yours did. I learn by chatting with plants."

"You do?"

"Yes. Don't you talk with plants?"

"Of course!" she confided with a wink. "But I don't tell my students that!"

"Why not?"

"Some of them wouldn't believe me."

"Listen, doña, have you ever heard of a healer called don Lucio?"

"Yes. I know him. He lives near Tlalnepantla. They call him 'the shaman.'"

"I have heard that he heals with plant spirits, that he does not use leaves or flowers. They say he invokes the plant spirits just by calling their names."

"I don't believe in that kind of thing. No, the blood of the plants is what heals. You've got to get it onto the body: the brain, the heart, the spine, the liver, the kidneys. You have to get the juice of the plants close to the important organs!"

After doña Modesta told me where to find him, I went to meet don Lucio myself. Arriving at his house, I found out that he was entertaining a Guatemalan herbalist and his two apprentices. They were all on their way to take the sheep to graze. I caught up with them in the road beside the corral. The old shaman had saddled his horse and was standing there holding the reins.

The Guatemalan herbalist was standing on tiptoes with a freshly picked plant in one hand. His other hand was cupped to his mouth. "And this?" he shouted into don Lucio's ear. "What do they call this plant in your language, in Nahuatl?"

Don Lucio pronounced the name.

The Guatemalan shouted back, "In Quiché, my language, we call this . . ." He made a softly guttural sound. "And here in Mexico, what medicinal use do you make of this plant?"

"I didn't know that this was medicinal!"

"Yes, *compadre,* this is medicinal!"

"Ah, imagine that! I had no idea! And what do you use it for?"

"This plant is good for old people when they are deaf like yourself," shouted the herbalist. "You let it dry in the sun for two or three hours, and then you stuff it in your ears."

"Oh, so this is medicinal!" said don Lucio good-naturedly.

We set out into the countryside with don Lucio on horseback, leading his sheep on a winding trail, and the Guatemalans and myself walking down the roadway. Whenever the herbalist saw a plant he recognized, he would stop, pick a stalk, and briefly explain to his students how to use it. Our progress was very slow; the teacher seemed to know everything that grew along the way. I was not privy to these lessons, as the three men spoke to each other in their own language.

Whenever don Lucio's path crossed our own, the teacher would accost him in Spanish.

"Compadre, what do you call this plant in Nahuatl?"

The apprentices would scribble down don Lucio's reply.

"Compadre, in Quiché we call this . . ." and the Guatemalan herbalist would make another soft, guttural sound. "And do you use this for food or medicine?" he would ask.

"No, I don't know any use for this."

"This is medicine, compadre! This is wonderful for . . . " and he would name an affliction.

"Oh, so this is a medicine, then! Imagine that! I had no idea!" The old man seemed to enjoy feigning ignorance as much as the younger one relished displaying his knowledge. Both of them seemed quite happy with themselves by the time we returned to don Lucio's home.

Don Lucio invited me into his parlor. The Guatemalans excused themselves, and I never saw them again.

The parlor was filled with the fragrance of freshly cut flowers. An entire wall was taken up by an elaborate altar filled with crucifixes, images of saints, and the like. The rest of the room was bare, save for five or six straight-backed chairs. The shaman motioned me to sit in one chair and took another next to mine.

He turned to me with a smile and clapped his hand on my knee. "Well, my boy, what can we do for you?"

"I do healing with plants," I said, "but I use the spirit of the plants, not the flesh." I put my hand on his forearm. "I understand you do something similar."

"What?" he said.

I cupped my hand to my mouth, leaned over close to his ear, and shouted, "I use plant spirits to heal people. You do too?"

"Yes! The spirits of the plants! That's it! Plants have movement! They have spirit! They even have soul! If not, they wouldn't be alive; the Lord wouldn't have put them here!"

"When you heal people, you don't make them eat or drink their medicine?"

"No! I do my work purely with intention!" He tapped his forehead with his index finger.

"There are very few of us who work that way," I said.

"Yes! Not like these people from Guatemala who go around looking for substances! This is the way I work. . . ." Here, don Lucio launched into a complicated story, using his free hand to touch mine at moments of particular interest. The gist of the story was how he used magical means to free a man he had never met from unjust imprisonment in a faraway city. After his release, the man traveled to don Lucio's village to offer thanks. The two men met by accident in the street. Don Lucio had no idea who the visitor was, but the visitor recognized him immediately. From his prison cell window, he had seen the shaman coming to his rescue.

"That's the way it is," the old man concluded. "That's the way it works."

"How did you learn what you know?" I asked him.

"No one taught me. When I was quite young, I was struck by lightning. I had walked out in the country by myself. I saw the lightning coming down at me. It was like a ball, all different colors, very beautiful! Then it hit me, and I lost consciousness. I was on the ground for more than two hours; it was no laughing matter! Then I got up and went home, but I was very sick. I would go into a coma, then come to for a few minutes, and then go back again. In all, I was in bed for three years. When my body was lying there, my soul was traveling and learning!

"The first year I spent with the Weather People in the heavens. I traveled all over the earth with the Weather People—to every country—bringing rain. The second year I spent with the Seeds. I met the spirit of all the plants that are cultivated by humankind. The third year I spent with the Flocks and the Herding People. I met all the different kinds of herding animals. I've been everywhere! I've seen it all! The Italians! The Eskimos! The Russians! The Africans! And you know, we are all brothers! You are my brother because the blood that flows in my veins also flows in yours! Isn't that so?"

"Yes, don Lucio, that's the way it is." We exchanged a glance. "You know, don Lucio, once when I was at the pyramid of El Tepozteco, I met the rain god." Intimidated by the Catholic images on his altar, I did not dare mention the god's pagan name.

"Tlaloc!" he said.

"Yes, Tlaloc! He taught me many things. I saw him with streams of water flowing from the palms of his hands."

"Of course! He's the one who hands out the water to this world. That's why I have him here with me. When it is dry and I ask for rain so that my people don't have to suffer, I have to have someone to back me up. So I keep Tlaloc with me."

"Wait a minute! You mean you have Tlaloc on your altar?"

"Naturally! Come, I'll show you." He took his hand off my knee and led me to the shrine.

Crowded among other religious images on the table, there stood a carved wooden mask of Jesus. Don Lucio removed the mask to reveal a grotesque stone idol of the Nahua rain god, Tlaloc.

We went back to our chairs and resumed our embrace. "How old do you think I am?" he asked.

Judging him to be about seventy-five, I said, "Oh, I don't know, maybe sixty-five."

"You didn't miss by much, my friend. I turned seventy-eight last September seventh. And yet, I still like the ladies! Now why do you suppose that is?" he grinned.

"Just natural, I suppose."

"Just natural, eh? Are you married, my boy?"

"Yes. I have children."

"Ah, I tell you my friend, this world is like no other. This is the only place you can make love and make lots of babies. The Lord wanted His people to be many, not just a puny few scattered here and there! That's why he made the world this way.

"But this world can be difficult, too. People do bad things to each other. Envy—it makes for a lot of illness, you know. It's terrible the things that people do to each other. Then I have to remove the illness people cause each other with their envy.

"This is not the only world, though. There is another world besides this one! The other world is beautiful, my brother! The food there is great! Not just tiny little bits like in this world; there you can eat huge amounts! You can make love all the time, and no babies! There is no fatigue! Your body is light like a feather! That world is beautiful. And that is where healing comes from. That's the way it is, brother, and that's how my work is: beautiful!"

"Thank you, don Lucio," I said. "It has been a real pleasure meeting you. I will come back and see you again soon. And if you ever find yourself in my town, my house is yours."

"Thank you. I will be waiting for your next visit. And when you return, bring me one of those American girls. A good one!"

When I returned, I brought no American girls, but don Lucio made no mention of it. He was busy preparing for a ceremony. A neo-Aztec group occupied his parlor: clouds of incense poured from the door and windows. Ceremonialists dressed in pre-Columbian costumes played lutes and sang in praise of the Star of Bethlehem and the Way of the Cross.

I entered the parlor. I was addressed by a bearded, athletic-looking man in a silver lamé loincloth and a three-foot-high plumed headdress. He asked me to remove my hat, which I did. I had heard this ceremony was to honor Tlaloc, so I had brought an offering of chocolate. I handed it to a priestess, who passed it through incense smoke, offered it to the four directions, and placed it at the altar among the other offerings, which were all flowers.

I walked outside to find don Lucio looking a trifle impatient.

"Where will your ceremony be held?" I asked.

"As soon as these people are done," he answered, "I will lead everyone to the church."

Obviously my intelligence had been wrong. This event could not be in honor of Tlaloc. No pagan god would be honored in a Catholic church. I wondered what kind of ceremony don Lucio would give. After a long wait, the old man picked up two baskets of flowers and set out toward the village church. I followed behind, lugging a heavy, five-foot candle he had asked me to carry.

The church was decorated with hundreds of candles, thousands of flowers, and lots of colored paper. It was the festival of La Candelaria: "Jesus, Light of the World." Scarcely had don Lucio placed his offerings before the altar when the Aztec troupe marched in with censors smoking. They placed themselves in formation before the altar and began to chant loudly. Village people started arriving. A contingent of young girls in luxurious, white first-communion dresses took their place next to the semi-naked Aztecs. The village priest walked up to the altar and put on his vestment.

Before long, a throng of faithful filled the church and spilled out onto the steps of the entrance. Mass was celebrated.

The Aztecs began a parting song. They backed out of the church with military precision, still singing and playing their instruments. By the time they got to the courtyard, the village brass band was already blaring a spicy tune, and skyrockets were exploding in booming clusters. Vendors were hawking candy and soft drinks. The girls in the white dresses flocked out, giggling. A couple of violinists sawed away at a dance tune, unheard in the din. It was the typical Mexican chaos, and nothing at all to do with Tlaloc—or so I thought. I left without saying goodbye to don Lucio.

I drove home under the usual clear blue skies, for it was the second of February—the height of the dry season. That night I was awakened by claps of thunder announcing a downpour. When I got up the next morning, the town was soaked, and the sky was faultlessly blue, promising many more weeks of sunny weather. I thought of don Lucio's altar, where the rain god stood hidden behind a mask of Jesus Christ.

chapter 20

PLANT SPIRIT HEALING IN WEST AFRICA

This interview showed me that plant spirit medicine is thriving in West Africa. Siri Gian Singh Khalsa spent several years in Togo researching a doctoral thesis on medical practices in that country. I visited him at his home in Sacramento, California, and asked him to share what he learned about the presence of plant spirit healing in Togo. He spoke about the interaction between traditional healers and Western doctors, and he described one remarkable healer in particular: Tobae Agbaga Asou.

Eliot: You went to West Africa, to Togo. How long ago?

Siri: I was there from 1980 to 1984. I was comparing the history of traditional medicine and Western medicine in Togo. Primarily I was focusing on the twentieth century. I tried to take my story as far back as I could go with the traditional healers.

Eliot: What did you discover about the role of herbs and plant spirits in traditional African healing?

Siri: The herbs were used in every facet of healing. There
          was a spirit associated with each herb that created the
          healing. Sounds were used to invoke those spirits in dif-
          ferent plants. They [the healers] also went into altered
          states through trance and sometimes through chemical
          means to have access to the information that the herbs
          could give them. Certain people had trained as long
          as twenty years in order to hear the spirits of the herbs
          talking to them.

Eliot: Is this something that has a long lineage?

Siri: Yes. A friend of mine, Dr. Merrick Posnansky, one of
          the premier archaeologists of Africa, has found that one
          of the best ways to find villages that were in existence
          six, seven, eight hundred years ago is to go anywhere
          in Africa and find where their herbs encircle something,
          then dig inside where those herbs grow—that would be
          the village. Many of the most widely used herbs would
          be grown secretly or openly around the village so that
          they [villagers] could have access to these really crucial
          plants. There are instances where we can prove that
          certain herbs were used thousands of years ago. Accord-
          ing to the traditions in the communities I studied, their
          herbal use goes back thousands of years.

Eliot: It is not necessarily the leaf or the root or the body of
          the plant that is used in the healing, but the spirit or
          essence of the plant. Is that right?

Siri: Yes, that is right! Each part of the plant had different
          qualities of spirit, and there was also an overall plant
          spirit. The healers paid attention to both. So bark from
          one plant would be used for one purpose and the flower
          for another purpose and the leaf for another purpose,
          just as Western botanists do.

Eliot: Do you have any stories to tell about healings that you saw specifically involving plant spirits?

Siri: Every time there was a healing there were plants involved. Each plant had to be communicated with in a specific way. Sounds of drums or voice would always be used to quicken the spirit of the plant. Something had to be done over the herbs in order to activate them and to make that herb an ally to the patient.

Eliot: Were you able to follow up on any cases?

Siri: Yes. Since I was studying with Western doctors and going to one of the most conservative institutions in the United States, the medical-history department at UCLA, I had to include Western opinions of what was happening. I had hundreds of interviews with Western doctors and thousands of interviews with traditional healers. The medical doctors would tell me about the illness of people they were treating. Many people who had been diagnosed and treated by Western doctors would let me accompany them to traditional healers. I would get to see what herbs were given and how they were administered.

What I found was that for people who had diabetes—and we don't cure diabetes in the West, we just control it—the herbs would be used to cure diabetes. When they would go back to the doctor, there would be no sign whatsoever of diabetes. Cancers, heart problems, a tremendous range of problems were diagnosed by the Western practitioners and then treated by the traditional practitioners. Sometimes I would have to pay the person to go back to the medical doctor. They felt that they were okay, so why would they waste their time? I wanted to have the validation by the physician, who sometimes would be very surprised.

The older doctors were Africans who had studied at the University of Paris Medical School or the University of Lyons Medical School in France. The younger MDs were very scathing and critical of the "superstitious, primitive, useless ways of the traditional healers." The older medical doctors who were African were always in respect of those ways because they had learned the limits of what they could do. They had seen that the African healers could cure things they [the medical doctors] could only hope to control at best—maybe kill the pain, but not to cure.

There developed a real interaction between the two systems. Everybody that I interviewed in this town would go to traditional healers first for certain things and the medical doctors for other things. None of the traditional healers I studied with could say they hadn't gone themselves or sent one of their family members to a Western doctor for certain things. They were tremendously open. They were always experimenting and always changing their system. It was more of a fluid system than the Western system was. All plants had spirits and powers, but also the earth, the air, the water, and all of nature.

Eliot: Tell me about the man you were closest to. What was his name?

Siri: His name was Tobae Agbaga Asou. He had a very interesting apprenticeship. He was taking a walk one day along a very rocky dirt road. An old man came up to him on a bike. It seemed amazing the old man could be riding a bike; there were so many rocks in the road. The man said, "Come back here tomorrow. I would like to show you something very important." Asou went back the next day, and again the old man appeared on a bike, but this time on a nearby hill where they could hear drumming. It was wonderful drumming—some kind of ceremony. The man went with him to the top of the hill where the ceremony was, and people seemed to recognize him. They hugged him [Asou] and were so happy to see him. He didn't recognize any of them. He was encouraged to stay there for a while, so he sat down. Then he felt a numbing in his body. He tried to get up but he couldn't move. He got very scared. The next thing he knew, he was going into the ground—deeper and deeper and deeper. He stayed there for nine earth years!

Eliot: In what he called the Underworld?

Siri: He went to the very center of the earth. In that place were the most gifted teachers he had ever met. Those teachers taught him about herbs, about invoking spirits of herbs, and various aspects of healing. There were several dozen people who came to the Underworld at the same time to learn healing. The ones who could read and write took notes, and the ones who couldn't were tested every night to make sure they remembered. My friend was one of the group that had to be tested.

I had interviewed many of his family members from the little village he lived in near Lomé, and they talked about how he had disappeared. They thought he had been killed by some animal. He [Asou] was gone for nine earth years. Those nine years in the Underworld were like centuries. He said it was a different time sense there. The amount that he learned and the number of days were many more than nine years of regular earth time. He learned lifetimes of information, particularly about the use of herbs. Then he came back, and there was great rejoicing, and he became a healer.

[Asou] was one of the most kind and bright and funny and empathic people I have met in my life. He had tremendous humility. He also had a very strong sense of self—tremendous personal power. He had about thirty apprentices, and about five hundred people came to his compound for healing every day—just wall-to-wall people.

Eliot: How did he minister to all those people?

Siri: His apprentices did some of the work. At any time
he had about thirty apprentices. [Asou] could look at
people and sense what they needed. I stayed with him
sometimes from two in the morning until two the next
morning. He would be with people nonstop. He would
tell his apprentices to prepare certain herbs for some
people. For others, he would tell them where to pick
certain herbs. Or he would give ceremonies to invoke
spirit, and the spirit would tell them what herbs to
use and how to activate the spirits of these herbs. He
treated everybody differently. With some people he
would be very funny, and they would be howling with
laughter. With other people he wouldn't say anything;
he would just listen. He might lecture and scream at
his patients until they would cry. It would be a rapid
succession of one group after another for at least twelve
hours straight. He would get up every morning at about
three-thirty and invoke different spirits of herbs and
do certain chants. He would work on himself or purify
himself for the work he had to do that day. Always the
herbs were central to what he did.

Eliot: You mentioned once that many of his apprentices were
well-respected healers in their own right.

Siri: Most of them had already achieved a high level of
renown in their own villages before they went to him to
study further about herbs. For [Asou] it wasn't simply
the herb as we know it in the West, but it was the
spirits associated with the herb. When you combine
different herbs, then it brings different spirits than the
spirits of the individual herbs.

Eliot: Would you recount the story of your extraordinary
contact with Asou and his plant spirits?

Siri: I like to get up early in the morning and do yoga. In Togo, I did yoga from three-thirty until six o'clock every morning. I would do yoga and meditate and pray. No one had seen what I did. I had been going to this healer about three times a week to get interviews and to observe healing.

Then after two or three months, [Asou] called me to him and said he felt very close to me and wanted to be friends, but he was in tremendous pain because he felt I had no idea who he really was. I couldn't understand who he was unless I could see and sense the spirits around him that were affecting him. Unless we know what powers are affecting a man, we can't really know who that man is. He would be happy to show me how to invoke plant spirits that would give me a vision of who he really was. So he asked me to come back in two weeks when he would have the proper herbs prepared.

He also told me that he had been "coming to my apartment" since I arrived in the country. He was with me the two and a half hours I exercised in the mornings, and he loved what I did. He told me in detail what he saw. He showed me some of the exercises I did—the kundalini yoga. He loved the kind of breathing I did. He loved the aroma of the flowers. He said they were very good for you. They were tuberoses. He said I had the wrong kind of incense and he would get me the correct incense. I was too limited in having just white candles; I needed seven different colors of candles.

Eliot: In the flesh, he had never been to your apartment?

Siri: That is correct. [Asou] had not been to my apartment in the flesh, nor had anybody else from his group. No one had been to my apartment for my morning spiritual practice. No one had been there except for my wife. Actually, I wasn't surprised that he knew all of that. I

felt closer to him. He knew so many details that I felt
he had been to my house in the mornings.

[Asou] had the herbs waiting when I came back two
weeks later. He could pick them out just perfectly with
these strong massive hands, although they were dry and
could crumble easily. The respect that he touched the
herbs with really impressed me. It touched me in a way
I hadn't been touched. Seeing his way of being with
them communicated something important to me. He
picked out three different herbs and told me to put all
three leaves under each of the seven candles, to burn
the incense he gave me while I did my usual two and
a half hours of meditation and yoga practices. He told
me some words to use at the end of my practices, to
invoke the spirits in the plants, which would call upon
his spirit.

When I did that, my wife and I were together. We
heard thunder and saw lightning in the room. We felt
vibration and the roaring of a large animal. It seemed
like a lion. In our minds' eyes, we saw crocodiles in the
room—both of us. I felt like [Asou] was in the room.
I was seeing him as I hadn't seen him before. He was
transparent. He let me go inside of his body. I felt pain
in his chest from smoking a lot. I felt the body was
ravaged by alcohol. But most of all, I felt the greatness
of the person. I had never known a human could be
so committed to continuously serving other people. I
never knew that a person could channel all the time,
as he seemed to do. I also felt contradictions in him—
pain in his body, dilemmas he was in. It was a very
plausible picture of a full human being that I got.

When I went back to him, I told him what I saw
and what I did. Then he confirmed that these animals
[the lion and crocodiles] were his protector animals.
They were very important to him. Yes, his chest did
hurt a lot. Nobody had told him he was smoking too
much. Everybody was afraid to tell him what he was

doing was wrong. He appreciated getting the feedback. The alcohol was terrible for his body in the quantities he had to consume, but the spirits who were linked to him wanted the alcohol. The only way they could get it was if he drank it. [Asou] would drink huge quantities every day. But whatever the reason for his drinking, he was a great man. He helped many people until his death last year.

chapter 21

GRANDMA BERTHA GROVE

I met Bertha Grove at her home on the Southern Ute Reservation one icy autumn morning in 1991. As she opened the door to her modest house and greeted me with a warm smile, I immediately understood why people call her Grandma. We went into her kitchen and unloaded the bags of groceries I had brought, and then she showed me into her parlor. She sat in an armchair beneath an enormous mounted buffalo head, and I installed myself in a sofa opposite her. Before she allowed me to switch on my tape recorder, she asked me to explain exactly what it was I wanted. I told her that I used the spirits of plants as medicine. I said that I thought it was important for people to know that plants have spirits that can heal, so I was writing a book about it, and I hoped that she would be willing to share some of her wisdom.

She seemed satisfied, and nodding for me to begin recording, she chanted a long prayer in the Ute language. The interview that followed was both deep and broad, for Grandma Bertha spoke almost until midday. I transcribe here the parts that have to do with plant spirit medicine.

Bertha: That's what I have to do when somebody comes asking me something like that—I have to say a prayer, have to ask the Grandfathers what you come looking for, what you want, because they know you, and they understand what it is that I have to tell you. I have to ask permission to say it; I don't just say it right off the bat.

It's the same way when we go gather the plants. There's different times and seasons to gather them. Some you can gather early in the morning, some at midday, some in the afternoon, and maybe the evening too. Some you gather at moonlight time, some in spring, some in summer, some in fall. Some of the things we pick up in the winter, like cedar. We don't just go over there and start choppin' or pickin'. When we go, we take tobacco or whatever gift that I'm going to give to them.

Supposing you're the cedar. It's just like I'm asking you a favor, asking for your help, asking for some of your clothing or your limbs. We tell you why we're going to use it, what we're going to do for people. When I say that and get the okay, then I give my gift. I usually tie a scarf. Whenever I see a sale, I usually buy some scarves; that way I have some all the time, and I keep them and some tobacco in my car, because you never know what plants I'm going to find.

Once you got your permission, you just take what you need. Never be greedy—that's one of the rules. If you need some, get what you need, and if you have to get some for [other] people, get that too. But you have to ask that you're going to take more than you're going to use, because you are going to give some to the people. And that's the way we do it. I don't know, is that the way you do things?

Eliot: Yes, yes.

Bertha: Supposing you're using the leaves or the branches or the stems. You make a tea or a poultice, and then what do you do with it after?

Eliot: I find that the main thing is to get the permission of the
           spirit that is going to help me help others. If I can make
           that relationship with the spirit of the plant, I don't
           need the leaf or the root or whatever. Sometimes I can
           ask the spirit of the plant to come through my hands.

Bertha: But you don't actually use the plant to make a tea?

Eliot: One of my main helpers is like a messenger, so I ask
           the messenger to bring the spirit of whatever plant that
           person needs.

Bertha: Like you say, everything has a spirit. The plants and
           trees and rocks are people, too. It's good the way you
           do things. I tell people it's good that they learn different
           ways of doing things. They can teach others, and I teach
           my way, and it's all to help heal people.

Eliot: How do you find out how a certain plant can help?

Bertha: Mostly it's your guardian spirit, your inner self, that
           tells you. You and I, we really don't know anything. It's
           the spirits that work through us; we're just the instru-
           ment these things work through. I have to ask the
           Creator to help me, and whatever way He tells me to do
           it, that's the way I'll move around. It might not be the
           same for different persons. Each person has their own
           body, mind, and spirit, and so the treatment is indi-
           vidual. It would be different for another person with
           the same ailment. It's the same when you talk to people;
           you have to treat them individually.

Eliot: Do you ever ask the spirits of the plants?

Bertha: That's what I'm asking for when I'm out there gathering
           the plant. I'm talking to the spirit of that plant. Have
           you seen them spirits?

Eliot: Yeah. Do the plants tell you how to use them?

Bertha: Uh-huh, they tell you. The spirit that you're talking
          about is universally in everything. That's why you have
          to have respect for animals and birds and plants. You
          know, even Mother Earth has got a lot of power in her.
          That's what I try to tell people: walk sacredly on Mother
          Earth. Mother Earth knows you—where you've been,
          where you're coming from. The spirits of everything are
          everywhere, surrounding us. You're watched by a thou-
          sand eyes every day, every move you make. So you ask
          permission when you're out there. You ask the Creator
          and you talk to Mother Earth and you talk to the Four
          Directions because you're using all of it. That plant
          did not come by itself. It came by Mother Earth. The
          sun came up and warmed it. The blessing is in there.
          The rain fell on it to make it grow, so you thank the
          Thunder Beings and the Cloud People for letting this
          plant grow. You thank the wind that blew, and you ask
          the Four Grandfathers and Grandmothers in the Four
          Directions for permission.

          This plant has spirit, and it didn't get spirit by itself.
          The Creator is the one who put it there. Anybody can
          use it; all you have to do is ask for help. You don't have
          to carry medicine bags around; just use what is in front
          of you. It's there to help people. It's got power: sticks,
          rocks, Mother Earth—even the wind has power. You
          can help people like that.

          Like you said, it can come through your hand.
          Your hand is the most powerful thing you have. It's
          used to help people, to bless people, so you can't hit
          anybody with it, right? But that's good you use your
          hands that way.

          Like I say, there's many ways of helping people—
          through the plants, the water. You can use anything
          in this world. Like the hair of that Grandfather. [She
          points to the buffalo head on the wall above her.] One

old Taos man gave me that for people who are going out of their mind. He said, "Keep it. One day you might use it." So different people have taught me—different tribes—you know.

Eliot: Could you talk a little more about how you learned?

Bertha: Oh, well, I grew up with my grandfather and he was a medicine man, one of the Ute. When a couple had more children than they could take care of in the old days, one was given to the grandparents or to the uncle or aunt. I was given to my grandparents, and they raised me. He [my grandfather] was a medicine man, and I grew up in that atmosphere. I grew up in a teepee, one of the last teepees on the reservation, so I know how to live in a teepee, how you're supposed to be in there, and how you're supposed to be with a medicine man. What I didn't understand until I was older was that to each of us—there were five that he had given the gift to—there was going to come a time when we would use it. I started dreaming, you know.

Eliot: How old were you?

Bertha: When it first began, I was still in my teens. This thing would talk to me, and I'd get scared. They told me, "The Creator chose you to do His work." And I made a prayer, and I said, "No, I'm too young. I can't do this work." So it kind of went away. Then I had kids; I had my children when I was real young.

Eliot: You prayed that this gift be taken away?

Bertha: Yeah, I was scared of it. So in my twenties, it came back again. I said, "I got kids to raise; I got no time for this. Wait till my hair turns gray." It said, "Okay." But in the meantime, people are coming to me telling me a lot of

189

things I should know—elderly people from different tribes. I'm not out there seeking for it; they're coming to me, and I'm learning. I'm seeing things in a gradual sort of way.

Well, in my early thirties, my hair turned gray. "You said, 'Wait till my hair turns gray,' and it's gray now!"—that's what that spirit told me. I said, "Wait a while." Then I got sick. I got asthma; I got crippled up with arthritis, couldn't walk, couldn't work any more. My husband said, "Maybe you ought to listen to what they tell you."

Then I started dreaming of [the] Sun Dance. I'd never seen women [do the] Sun Dance, but I'd helped my husband and my boys into the Sun Dance ceremony, 'cause my grandfather that raised me was a Sun Dance chief. I'd been helping him since I was a little girl. They made me do things that was teaching me, I guess. I thought I was being treated mean . . . the hardships I had in my childhood . . .

I used to herd sheep when I was little, you know. Way out there in the hills, all by myself, with just my dog and the sheep. You know, you sit out there in the hills, and you're wondering about everything. That was part of the stuff that I was supposed to learn—observing nature, the plants. I was talking to them because I had nobody else to talk to. I'd see them rocks, pick them up, talk to them, put them back. They were my playmates. Flowers, rocks, and brush and whatever were my playmates. I didn't realize I was being taught.

I started Sun Dancing. One day I had a dream that said, "Now's the time." I'd worked for the BIA [Bureau of Indian Affairs] for so long, I said, "I can't just up and quit." But the dream told me I had to quit now, take them white man's shoes off, put on moccasins. For four years, I wore those moccasins through spring and fall, summer and winter, because the spirit told me I could never put no shoes on. Then I went Sun Dancing, and that's where my physical body began to come back into shape again. I couldn't get up by myself, but my husband came over early to the arbor where we were dancing, and I was already up, and he said, "How did you get up?" "I got up," I said.

You know, that asthma went away. I always tell people I'm a testament to what plants can do for you, what spirits can do for you, what faith can do for you. At my age—I'm almost seventy—I can move faster than most younger ones. I can get up, walk a long ways, take care of our house, cook for us, which I'm grateful for.

I was trained for who and what I was, and I knew why those old people had been showing me. It all came together little by little. One old man, he's from the Northern Utes, he helped me a lot, made me understand about the spirits. And I have another from up there, he taught me a lot about the spirits, the Grandfathers, the Grandmothers, about the sweat lodges. Some of it I learned through Sun Dancing and through my vision quests.

The way I see it, everything is good; the Creator said He made everything good, and it's still the same way. It is just man that thinks, "That plant is no good; that animal is no good." There is a reason for Him creating it. There is a reason for snakes, for flies. We say spray the heck out of them, but I found out if you talk to them they won't bother you any more.

These spirits are real. If you believe in them, they'll help you. That is what those medical doctors don't understand. They could do a lot of things if they could just believe in this Creation, in the spirits. Maybe there are a few who know that, but very few. Even in our own clinic they think we're crazy if we talk about that. Lot of people think you're crazy if you do things like that. I guess you come up against that.

Eliot: I usually don't tell people that the spirits are helping. Maybe they wouldn't be there if they knew.

Bertha: It doesn't bother me what people think, because I've
          had my experiences. I was told, "Never mind if people
          laugh at you, call you names. Don't worry about that.
          You do My work for me. I'm the one you'd better be
          scared of; I'm the one that's making you do this work,
          helping you." So that's what I do—is follow the Creator.
          If somebody asks me for help, I pray about it first. If
          I'm supposed to help, I will. If I'm not, then I'll get
          somebody else.

Eliot: Your dreams, are they nighttime dreams or daytime dreams?

Bertha: Whenever I sleep. If they're nighttime dreams, then I
          wake up [afterward]. Sometimes they're daytime dreams.
          You think you're dreaming, but you're not. If it's quiet,
          I can meditate or I'm doing something, but I'm like
          dreaming, seeing things. Sometimes I can close my eyes
          and talk real quiet, and I can see. If I go to a ceremony,
          I can talk to Grandfather Fire; I can talk to the Grand-
          fathers, and they'll show me. It's like a TV there.
              These things don't lie, you know. People can lie, but
          the Creation can't lie. So if a plant spirit is talking to
          you and you're absorbing it, then you do what it tells
          you to do. You don't go beyond, adding little fringes to
          it, or something like that. Maybe someone expects you
          to do more, but it's like, "This is what I'm supposed to
          do, and that's it." That's all.

Eliot: Could you talk about when you healed somebody using
          a plant?

Bertha: Okay . . . Let's see, there are so many . . . okay, I'm
          going to leave some parts out, just tell you other parts.
              One time there was this family in Taos, and this
          lady's uncle was having a hard time, because somebody
          burnt down his house and his trading post. Well, about
          two, three years before we'd been down there, and

she [the lady] called me "Mother," you know. She took me to see her uncle at his trading post; we didn't know him then. She introduced us, and he gave me a shawl out of his store, a red-and-blue shawl for one of the ceremonies that we have. There's stories behind that, too. He gave my husband a gourd, my friend a feather—different stuff like that. So we thanked him.

So years later, he's having a problem, and they told us to come down there and do a ceremony for him. So my husband and I took off. I'm driving over Tres Piedras, up that big mountain. When I got way on top, all of a sudden something tells me, "Turn around!" So, quick, I turned around and stopped. There's this aspen tree, and I told my husband, "I'm supposed to get something here." He said, "Okay." That's one thing about him, he never questions. So we got out, and I told him, "We need four branches, four twigs from the top of the tree."

Eliot: The tree told you that?

Bertha: Yes. See, I don't know why I'm doing this; I'm just doing what the tree is telling me. So my husband is hanging up there, and the grandchildren are laughing: "Hey, Grandpa is like a monkey!" So he pulls the branches over to me, and I cut them off and do my prayers. I put water on the towel I carry with me, and I wrap it away. I don't know what I'm going to do with it.

So we get down there into Taos, and they're having the ceremony, and the branches are still in the van. Then, after midnight, "Hey, that plant is talking again!" So I tell my husband, "Go get that plant for me," and he went and got it. I'm just doing what the branches are telling me, so I go up to these people I don't know and I say, "You Taos people use aspen in your ceremonies, your feasts, your kivas, and at this time, I'm going to ask you to use these aspen branches to help that person standing over there. Use this; bless him with it." They said, "All right," and got everything situated.

At that time I didn't know that man. I didn't know that he was the uncle of the person we were doing the ceremony for. I didn't know that this man didn't like his nephew and that he did him wrong. All I knew was the plant is telling me to give it to that man. And he gets up there, and he starts to pray. He's talking in his own language, but the ladies told me the next morning, they said, "How did you know? How did you know he was the one who burned down his house and store?" I said, "I didn't know. I was just doing what the plant was telling me to do." They told me that in his prayer he was confessing, that he was sorry that he had hurt him like that.

He told me the next morning, "When I was touched by that branch, it was so powerful. The energy just come and shook me, and I wanted to scream or howl, but I held myself. I could feel that force. It made me tremble like a lightning strike or something."

I told the man who was blessing him, "You keep it, and sometime before three days are over, you take it back up on that mountain where nobody goes around, and you thank it for the blessing you got."

The next morning that uncle was trying to make him give the branches to him, saying, "I'll put it in the kiva; it's really powerful." But I told him, "It's not going to do anything unless the spirit is with it. It won't do anything unless you're doing what it tells you to do. The plant said it came through here, and now it's got to go up there, up in the mountains, back where it belongs."

And that man who the ceremony was for, he got all right—built another store, he became the war chief, became governor. He's doing all right, see?

That's what that plant can do for you: make a way for you like that. You just have to keep your mind, your heart, your spirit open to the Creation so you can hear these things.

So that was one time that we helped with aspen leaves. Sometimes I use sage.

Eliot: Do you have a good sage story?

Bertha: Lots of things I do, I don't remember them. You're not supposed to, I guess; you just do it. . . . Let's see, a sage story.

We were on our way to Utah one time, and I said, "Stop!" I told my husband, "Over there; pick four of them, just four." So he did.

Eliot: This is sage?

Bertha: Yes, four of those little sages. We took that sage—where we were going was to another ceremony this lady was having for herself.

Eliot: Was she ill?

Bertha: She was ill; she was diabetic. Her legs were swelling up so that she couldn't walk. So I told them: "Use that sage on her." So by morning her leg was normal size. She got up and walked out. You just rub it; you kind of press it on her.

There's a lot of ways to help people, lots of ways. Sometimes we put it on a patient and blow into it. Peppermint is good that way too.

Eliot: How do you mean, blow into it?

Bertha: What I do is I dip it [the sage or peppermint] in running water four times and ask the Creation, Four Directions, and Mother Earth. Before you put it in the water, ask Grandmother Water for help. You're asking everything to support that Grandmother. That's a Grandmother too, that female sage. That one is real pretty. You just put it on [the patient's skin] and blow into it.

Sometimes when I use the sage like that, I take out whatever is in there—the pain. You'd be amazed what you'd find, some of the things that people do to each other. Maybe you'd know, maybe you don't. They call it witchcraft. You can take that out, too.

See, the Creation and the Four Directions, they're real powerful and they're supporting that sage, and you're supporting it too, with your breath, because you are a spirit, too. All spirits have to work together—the spirit of the plants and everything. Sometimes you need support, and even that plant needs the support of the Mother Earth where it came from. So you learn. You're learning. Maybe you have learned more than me.

But like I say, I'm not just a plant [healer], I'm the whole thing, the whole Creation.

The Grandfather, he's the one you have to talk to, the one you have to ask, because he's the Creator, and you always have to ask his permission . . . to use the spirit of this plant here. Then you gotta thank the spirit of the plant. Then you gotta thank the Creator and Mother Earth where it comes from. You gotta learn to be appreciative of things.

Do you see them plant spirits around you?

Eliot: When I close my eyes and relax. Usually I use drumming to help me; then I can see the spirits.

Bertha: Yeah, that's what we do in our ceremonies. Someone is drumming. That's good, you know.

Once you begin to know the spirits, you begin to put things in their place, as time comes along. . . .

We use the sage for smudging a lot, for blessing. It helps clean out the things from around you that block your spirit. Do you do anything besides talking to the spirits when you're helping people? Do you go through some formalities?

Eliot: Not usually. When you're dealing with white people in the city, you start to do those things and . . .

Bertha: You can't do anything the way they understand.

Eliot: So the other things I keep to myself.

Bertha: That's good. I'm glad you do that. I got to do that, too, with my white people. *[Laughs.]* I got to learn to do it like that when I work with white people.

Eliot: Well, people who come to you are open minded.

Bertha: Yeah, a lot of times I'll give them a brief explanation of why I'm using this, why I'm doing this. That way they can have a little bit of understanding of it.
           I'm glad you're working in that way. That's a new thing. See, I learned from you. I'm going to put that into practice! We ask the spirit, but asking the plant to do the work [of collecting and delivering the medicine], hey, that takes a lot off me! *[Laughs.]* Make it work, make the plant work, instead of me doing it!
           Anyway, I'm glad to meet you. I hope I told you what you wanted to know.

Eliot: This has been wonderful!

Bertha: Like I say, the plants was human one time, and they gave their life, their spirits, because we're asking them for help. It's just like the food we eat. It was alive; one time it was moving around, and it gave up. That's why I tell them when you go hunting, you have to talk to the spirit of the wild animals, thank them, because they

197

gave their lives. Even that fire: that tree [whose trunk you are burning] was a living thing, was growing. So when you build a fire, think about it. It gave its life so you could have heat. Even the coal, gas, butane, came out of Mother Earth; it's part of her. Even the water you drink. People don't look at it like that. That's why people contaminate it. They don't understand. "The Water of Life," that's what the Indians call it. We have great respect for it. I learned from experience, so I go back and say thank you. The Water of Life—some of it comes from within the Mother Earth, but, hey, government is taking it all away from us. They're even in the underground waters now.

My grandfather told me, "Way down the line, they're gonna be fighting over water. You keep your Indian way of life. Maybe you can save some of your people that way, when the time comes. I'm not going to be around, but these ways might help you save yourself and some of your people when the time comes."

A lot of people wonder why I talk to people like you. They say I'm giving away knowledge of Indian people. But there's lots of Indian people that's trying to share our beliefs with people of other cultures so that you can understand me and I can understand you. If we don't include the spiritual part, then we can't understand each other.

You have your culture. They used plants, too—way back. In European countries, they had the knowledge of the plants. So I tell people, "You have it, too. This isn't just my secret or Indians' secret. You have a right to know, because you had it, too. It's just that somewhere along the line it got lost. You just need to recapture it, and when you do, we'll get along."

Eliot: It's so important to start learning from Mother Earth again.

Bertha: Uh-huh, I learned a long time ago about owning things.
Pretty soon they own you. You gotta make payments.
So a lot of people are going back to a simple way of
living. Because really, we make it hard for ourselves.
That's what one old man told me, "There's nothing
to life." He said, "Sun comes up, we get up, do our
prayers, and we eat breakfast. Through the day we do
what we have to do—go visit people or go work. Then
evening comes, sun goes down, we come back home,
eat again, talk. Whatever we done all through the day,
we talk about it. Then we go to bed, make our prayers
again, sleep. Then the sun comes up, we do it again, go
through life. We make it hard for our own self 'cause
we put in all these worries. We make our own problems. But it's really simple. You just live. Enjoy yourself."
That's what he told me.

He was right. I live that way now. I'm not in a hurry.
I don't rush around. Frustration, hate, bitterness will
take a physical toll on you. That's what's gonna make
you sick. Cancer, tumors, diabetes is caused by all
these things you put on your own self. Heart trouble,
stroke—hate and bitterness causes strain on your heart.
Don't do it. It doesn't matter what anybody says—that's
their problem. Don't carry it.

Now I just say, "Grandfather, take care of it, whatever's not right."

Us Indians don't have no devil or hell. It isn't that
way. It's just our thoughts that make it that way. The
way I'm telling you is the way I was taught, the way
I was shown. I could sit back here and make up lies,
stories about the plants, the miracles I've done. But
it wasn't that way. You would believe me, 'cause I'm
an elder, but I can't do it that way. I have to tell the
truth the way I've experienced it. If I lie to you, I have
to answer to that Person up there. That's one I'm very
respectful of, very fearful of what that would do. If you
lie, you have to live with it. In time it's going to affect

your mind and your body, so why lie? So you be yourself, that's what I tell people. That's what I tell you.

I hope I have been of help to you, a little bit anyway. I've done something in the name of the Creation, the Grandfathers, and the plants—on their behalf.

You have gone a long way into the plant things. Even herbalists don't go that far. They just use it like giving you an aspirin. They give you a capsule, but they really haven't gone to that spirit. But you have. You have that messenger. That's something for me to think about. I have learned something from you, and I appreciate it. As time goes on, I'll think about it, and say, "That's what he was talking about."

That's about all I could say to you. I want to thank you for coming. In talking to you, I help myself. It's not very often I come across people who have the power and the energy to do this kind of work with the spirits.

Eliot: I think it's that most people don't have the interest.

Bertha: Maybe that's why. You have that knowledge; you'll go on with this. "Don't get too proud," I tell people. "Don't be getting in front of people. Stay back. Be humble."

conclusion

COMMUNITY
AND RITUAL

In the chapters on Fire, Earth, Metal, Water, and Wood, there are stories of men and women who became out of balance with the Five Elements. We saw how imbalance affected their lives and how they changed when balance was restored.

Each chapter also looked beyond the individual cases to see how we as a society are doing with respect to these five sacred forces. The record here is dismal. Individuality, selfishness, disrespect, fear, and aggression are rewarded and reinforced at every turn. Since we all necessarily live in society, no one is immune from these influences. Under the circumstances, it is miraculous that plant spirits help us so much. But when we consider the wellbeing of our communities, we reach the border between what the spirits can do for us and what we must do for each other.

A society that insists on uncontrolled growth will be cancerous. A people who disregard warmth and connection will have heart disease. In a world where it is not important to take care of each other, a few will be obese while many suffer from malnutrition. Where fear is promoted, violent death will follow. When nothing is sacred, almost anything can go wrong.

In chapter 2, the young man who worked as a gardener found his hay fever wonderfully improved after his first few plant spirit medicine sessions. On the other hand, we are experiencing widespread food allergies that plant spirit medicine often does not touch. What's the difference? The symptoms of the young gardener expressed an imbalance that was mostly personal. It is relatively easy for the plant spirits to rebalance a single individual, but when the whole society is out of balance, it's a different story. The current epidemic of wheat allergies, for example, is not so much a personal problem, but a societal one.

The sacred stories tell us that before the world began, some divine beings who would later become plants offered a deal to other divine beings who would later become humans. A few plant people agreed to undergo domestication in order to nourish and support the life of human people. In return, the plant people asked to be grown, prepared, and eaten with respect, dignity, and gratitude. The human people agreed to the deal and promised to abide by the terms.

In the case of wheat (and several other food plants), we have not kept our part of the bargain. Hybridization, genetic engineering, toxic chemicals—has anyone bothered to ask wheat how it feels about these things? The wheat people asked for certain demonstrations of respect and gratitude. Are offerings being given and traditional ceremonies performed in the corporate laboratories and boardrooms?

We've been treating this sacred gift of wheat as if we could do anything to it that would bring profit. Now the consequences are coming home to roost. The plant who agreed to be the staff of life for the peoples of the Middle East is now making people ill worldwide. The consequences don't necessarily fall on individuals who have been particularly disrespectful. When society is out of balance, the symptoms can show up on anyone.

Individual treatment won't go very far in solving this problem; instead, we will have to work together. Somehow the Metal of the community must be rebalanced, for Metal connects us to honor, value, and respect. It's not that wheat is sadistically having fun at our expense. On the contrary, the wheat spirit is still helpful. It is patiently showing us that a balanced community is needed in order for individuals to have good health and a good life.

These days people are encouraged to feel that the city limits of their community is their own skin. "It's all about you, baby!" Some people have a sense of community extending beyond themselves to the people in their family, neighborhood, or town. But almost nobody considers the nonhumans who live around them: the plants, animals, soil, waters, rocks, and sun. And only rarely does anyone realize that the Ancestors who came before us and the generations to come after are also community members—perhaps the most important community members of all.

Yes, community is meant to provide for you, but after your life is over, then what? Naturally, we hope the loved ones who survive us may live well, and to live well they need good relationships with others, human and nonhuman alike. How can we be in good relationship? The Ancestors have thousands of years of hard-won experience in this matter, and they would enjoy nothing more than to share it with you.

A functional community sees this as its first duty: to provide a good life for generations to come by following the wisdom of generations past. So no, it's *not* all about you, baby. A community engagement that provides for only you is nothing more than a brief indulgence. Community is about sustainability, and sustainability is not over when you are.

I feel at a disadvantage in this writing. I was as thoroughly steeped in individualism as just about anyone, and for all my experimentation with life in communes and ashrams, I myself have never had the good fortune to live in a viable community. Only now as I enter old age do I have a vision of community and the commitment to work towards it. But newcomer that I am, I take courage to speak from my experiences with the Huichol people and plant spirit medicine.

As one of the original First Peoples, the Huichols have been living in their homelands since the beginnings of humanity. Despite being hard pressed by the dominant society, today Huichol communities in the Sierra Nevada are vibrant. The people are clear that their success is due to staying true to their ancestral ways. Newborns are welcomed and named in baptismal rites. Adolescents are ritually initiated into womanhood and manhood. Elders are honored and consulted for wise counsel. The dead are given funerary rites to help them in their passage to the land of the ancestors. Corn is honored with a series of elaborate seasonal rituals. People make pilgrimages to sacred places of the sun, earth, growth, wind, fire, rain, peyote, springs, ocean, and mountains. At those places they give offerings, prayers, and songs; in return they receive health, knowledge, and special capacities. Civic matters are discussed and decided at well-attended community meetings. And throughout all of this is the presence of the shamans, who watch over the balance of the community, guiding the rituals, singing the instructions of the gods, and providing healing.

At one point I led a group to a Huichol village, a place where most visitors see poverty. An older Huichol woman asked, "Where are these people from?"

"Most are from the United States."

"Oh, those poor, poor people. If they are going to survive, they will have to go back to the past. And when they do, here we will be."

The Huichols' commitment to maintaining and preserving their gifts is practical; their gifts have worked well for a very long time. I'm sure the old woman was right. When our technology collapses, we won't look so impressive any more. If we have the good sense to get back to what really sustains people, we'll discover the Huichols, still planting corn with prayers and digging sticks.

My Huichol experience changed my attitude toward the future of plant spirit medicine. In the beginning, I felt the medicine was something *I* had discovered or developed. It was good, it was helpful, and I told myself I would share it with people if they were interested. I gave hardly a thought to the survival of the practice, but had you asked me about it then, I probably would have said something like, "If it survives, fine. If not, somebody else will come up with something good some other time."

I feel differently now. Plant spirit medicine was given by the plant spirits, the elemental forces, and the ancestors—not to me, but to you and others in need of healing or spiritual discovery. Surely there will be those who can benefit from it after I am gone, so the gift deserves to be honored and protected.

To this end, I am developing an outstanding faculty to succeed me as a teacher of plant spirit medicine. To this end also, plant spirit medicine has been given a home at the Blue Deer Center, a beautiful retreat center on sacred ground in New York State's Catskill Mountains. It is a home to feel at home in, not only because of the exuberance of the plant life there, but also because the Center's mission is to make available many ancestral teachings and practices that promote balance with the natural world.

Courses to train plant spirit medicine healers have been lengthened and strengthened, and continuing education for graduates is now required. Short courses for those interested in plant spirit medicine as a spiritual exploration and discovery have also been introduced.

Three organizations help support and legitimize the work: the Plant Spirit Medicine Association, the Plant Spirit Medicine Seminary, and the

Temple of Sacred Fire Healing. In former years I scoffed at such things, but no more. If the medicine is to live in this society, people must be able to trust that a plant spirit medicine healer with a certificate on the wall is a person who has completed rigorous training, has demonstrated competence, is committed to high ethical standards, and continues to learn and grow.

I'd also like to speak of my experience with the Sacred Fire Community. This is not a community in the usual sense of a group of people who live together in the same location. It is an international organization of people who gather around small, local hearths as our ancestors did. Guided by initiated fire-keepers who hold a modest ritual space, there is talk, laughter, song, and at times conflict and resolution. People rediscover what the Ancestors knew: the fire of the heart breaks down isolation and melts fear, and meeting with others in community around the fire brings meaning, purpose, joy, and self-knowledge to our lives. People share their concerns and their discoveries, but there is no doctrine or particular spiritual path that must be followed. Community gatherings provide a safe space for exploration.

As the exploration unfolds, Western people are remembering some of the things the Huichols and others never forgot. We are not solitary by nature. Our lives are played out together, in community, and community is not simply a matter of logistics. Community identifies our gifts and gives a place for those gifts to be received and appreciated. In this way, we come to know ourselves not as isolated units moving randomly in what seems to be a meaningless world, but as well-loved members of a warm and vital family that starts with our parents, brothers, and sisters, moves out to extended family and friends, then moves on to the entire village, and from there expands into the fantastic and diverse natural world, whose mountains and deserts, streams and forests, plants and animals are all affectionately known as Grandmothers and Grandfathers. When our lives are over, community escorts us to visit the Ancestors for a while; then community is there to welcome us back on our return.

No, community is not simply about logistics. It is more about creating a place where people feel related to everything. How does community work this magic? Through ritual. There can be no true community without it.

Do not mistake effective ritual for an empty ceremony, which is a pattern of acts that everyone is familiar with, yawns through, and is unchanged by. Ritual produces a living spiritual chemistry that changes everything. The young person enters initiation camp as a child, a person who is rightfully at the breast of the community. He or she emerges as a young adult, someone who has now *become* the breast of the community. To put it another way, the caterpillar has become a butterfly. The ritual produces that radical transformation.

My experience with plant spirit medicine showed me that when the conditions are right, the Divine restores long-forgotten ancestral practices. This still goes on today. The Sacred Fire Community has brought back initiation into adulthood, effective funerary rites, men's and women's retreats, and explorations of prayer and birthing practices. Local indigenous traditions are being exhumed and revived. In other words, the lost pieces of effective community are being put back into the puzzle. In the face of escalating violence and destruction, this is what gives me peace and confidence in a rich and joyous human future.

notes

1. For an in-depth look at this process, see Allan Savory's profound and fascinating book, *Holistic Resource Management* (Washington, DC: Island Press, 1988).

2. In the Five Element perspective, sympathy is in itself an emotion. You could say it is empathy—the capacity to feel what others feel—combined with the desire to bring comfort and relief to someone's discomfort and suffering.

3. Several months later, I introduced Charlotte and her class to a plant known as bleeding heart. We made a dream journey to meet the spirit of the plant. Afterward, she told me I must have given her bleeding heart in her first treatment, because the spirit she met was clearly the same one that came to her at that time. I consulted my treatment notes. She was right.

4. Charlotte's dream vision of her heart protector corroborated my assessment of her condition at the time she came for treatment.

5. Originally reprinted courtesy of the Sun Valley Center for the Arts and Humanities. From Fred Coyote, *I Will Die an Indian* (Sun Valley, ID: Institute of the American West, 1980).

6. Since initiation is a growth process powered by the Wood element, it is fascinating to note that the first instructor on a vision quest is often a tree spirit. Two recent accounts of this phenomenon come to mind: the initiation of Ron Geyshick, a Lac La Croix Ojibway healer (see *Te Bwe Win*, Toronto:

Summerhill Press, 1989), and that of Malidoma Patrice Somé,
a Dagara shaman from West Africa (see *Of Water and the Spirit,*
New York: Penguin, 1995).

resources

The **Plant Spirit Medicine Association** (plantspiritmedicine.org) offers information about plant spirit medicine, a directory of qualified healers, and a catalogue of upcoming courses, workshops, and other events.

The **Plant Spirit Medicine Seminary** (plantspiritmedicine.org/study/seminary) is a training facility of the Temple of Sacred Fire Healing, a nonprofit spiritual organization dedicated to spiritual healing training and practice.

The **Blue Deer Center** (bluedeer.org, 845-586-3225) is the headquarters for plant spirit medicine and an important home for traditional teachings and practices of heart. Contact the Center for information on all aspects of Eliot Cowan's work, as well as the offerings of other traditional healers, teachers, and ceremonial leaders.

The **Sacred Fire Community** (sacredfirecommunity.org) offers community fire gatherings, initiations for young women and young men, plus other programs for the cycles of life.

The **Sacred Fire Foundation** (sacredfirefoundation.org) provides funds for the survival and development of ancient wisdom and indigenous peoples. Its educational outreach includes *Sacred Fire* magazine and Ancient Wisdom Rising, a gathering of wisdom teachers.

about the author

Eliot Cowan was born in 1946 and was raised in Chicago, Winnipeg, and San Francisco. He graduated with a degree in anthropology from Pomona College and did postgraduate studies in ethnographic documentary filmmaking at UCLA.

Eliot began to study and practice herbalism in 1969 and set it aside after a few years to study acupuncture. Under the guidance of Professor J. R. Worsley, he received his licentiate, bachelor, and master of acupuncture degrees from the College of Traditional Acupuncture, Leamington Spa, England, and served on the faculty of that institution from 1979 to 1980.

In the early 1980s, Eliot once again turned his attention to herbal healing. This time he was instructed directly by the spirits of the herbs. Together with his plant mentors, he rediscovered the ancient practice of plant spirit medicine.

He apprenticed with the late don Guadalupe González Ríos, an elder Huichol Indian shaman. His graduation formalities were conducted in Mexico in 1997. In 1998, don Guadalupe ritually initiated Eliot as a teacher of shamanic apprentices. A second initiation was given five years later.

Having returned to the United States to live, Eliot devotes his time to the teaching and practice of plant spirit medicine, Huichol shamanism, and other ways of promoting Divine connection among our people.

about sounds true

Sounds True is a multimedia publisher whose mission is to inspire and support personal transformation and spiritual awakening. Founded in 1985 and located in Boulder, Colorado, we work with many of the leading spiritual teachers, thinkers, healers, and visionary artists of our time. We strive with every title to preserve the essential "living wisdom" of the author or artist. It is our goal to create products that not only provide information to a reader or listener, but that also embody the quality of a wisdom transmission.

For those seeking genuine transformation, Sounds True is your trusted partner. At SoundsTrue.com you will find a wealth of free resources to support your journey, including exclusive weekly audio interviews, free downloads, interactive learning tools, and other special savings on all our titles.

To learn more, please visit SoundsTrue.com/bonus/free_gifts or call us toll free at 800-333-9185.

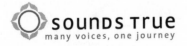

SOUNDS TRUE
many voices, one journey